The Anabolic Solution™

The Definitive Metabolic Diet, Training, and Nutritional Supplement Book for Recreational and Competitive Bodybuilders

By Mauro G. Di Pasquale, B.Sc., M.D., M.R.O., M.F.S.

Table of Contents

About The Author

I am presently a licensed physician in Ontario, Canada, specializing in Nutrition and Sports Medicine.

I hold an honors degree in biological science, majoring in molecular biochemistry and genetics (1968), and a medical degree (1971) – both from the University of Toronto. I am certified as a Medical Review Officer (MRO) by the Medical Review Officer Certification Council (MROCC), and as a Master of Fitness Sciences (MFS) by the International Sports Sciences Association (ISSA). I am also a member of the American Academy of Sports Medicine.

I was an assistant professor at the University of Toronto for ten years (1988 to 1998) teaching and researching athletic performance, nutritional supplements and drug use in sports.

I was a world-class athlete for over twenty years, winning the world championships in Powerlifting in 1976, and the World Games in the sport of Powerlifting in 1981. I was Canadian champion eight times, Pan American champion twice, and North American champion twice. I was the first Canadian Powerlifter to become a World Champion and first Canadian Powerlifter to total 10 times bodyweight in any weight class and I am the only Canadian to ever total ten times bodyweight in two weight classes.

Over the last four decades I have had extensive exposure to athletic injuries and disabilities, and ergogenic and nutritional supplement use by athletes. I have been chairman/member of several national and international powerlifting, bodybuilding and Olympic weight lifting sports federation medical committees. Over this period of time I have acted as a consultant, medical advisor, drug testing officer and technical expert on the pharmacology and pathophysiology of sports, nutritional supplement use and drug testing.

I was the Medical Director to World Wrestling Federation (now known as World Wrestling Entertainment) and World Bodybuilding Federation (WBF) and the acting MRO for the National Association for Stock Car Auto Racing (NASCAR).

At present I am the President of the International United Powerlifting Federation and the Pan American (North, Central and South America, Bermuda, the Bahamas and the Caribbean Islands) Powerlifting Federation.

I have written several books dealing with diet, nutritional supplements and the use of ergogenic aids by athletes. In 1995 I wrote two books. One of these books, the *Bodybuilding*

Supplement Review is a review of nutritional supplements and the other, the *Anabolic Diet*, was an attempt at setting up a working high fat, low carb diet for bodybuilders.

In 1997 I wrote *Amino Acids and Proteins for the Athlete – The Anabolic Edge* published by CRC Press was released in October 1997. I have also written and am in the process of writing chapters for several books on nutrition, sports medicine, substance abuse, fitness and weight training. At present I am working on several other books including a comprehensive nutritional supplement manual.

In the past thirty-five years I have written several hundred articles on training, diet, nutritional supplements, and drug use in sports for many magazines and association journals. I have written for and had regular monthly columns in all the popular bodybuilding and fitness journals including Muscle and Fitness, Flex, Men's Fitness, Shape, Muscle Media, Muscle Mag International, IronMan, Powerlifting USA and many smaller publications.

From 1996 to 1999 I was involved in writing, research and product development for Experimental and Applied Sciences (EAS) and Muscle Media, and was a member of the EAS Scientific Advisory Panel.

I have contributed chapters on diet and nutritional supplements to several fitness, weight and sports medicine books as well as books on anabolic steroids and substance abuse. The latest chapters on nutrition appear in *Energy-Yielding Macronutrients and Energy Metabolism in Sports Nutrition and in Nutritional Applications in Exercise and Sport*, both edited by Judy A. Driskell and Ira Wolinsky and published in 2000 and 2001 respectively by CRC Press.

I am in the process of finishing the nutritional, nutritional supplement and ergogenic aids section (about half the book) in the second edition of *Serious Strength Training* scheduled to be released this coming Spring by Human Kinetics.

In the past three decades I have been on several Editorial Boards for various fitness and strength magazines and was the Editor-in-Chief of a two quarterly international newsletter on sports nutrition and ergogenic aids.

I act as an international consultant for amateur and professional athletes and sports bodies on all aspects of training, nutrition and supplementation. I act as an international consultant and expert witness for amateur and professional athletes and sports bodies, private corporations and companies, and government agencies on legal matters relating to nutritional supplements, and the use and abuse, and drug testing of anabolic steroids, growth hormone and other ergogenic drugs.

I hold seminars and lecture all over the world on diet, nutritional supplements and training. In the past I have lectured and held seminars in dozens of cities in North America, and all over the world. I also formulate engineered, cutting edge, scientifically validated nutritional supplements for various companies that are sold under their specific labels. Most recently I formulated a new group of nutritional supplements meant to combat nighttime post absorptive catabolism and enhance the anabolic and recuperative effects of sleep. I am now working with several prominent researchers from the US and several other countries. Those in the US include doctors at Harvard Medical School and the Massachusetts College of Pharmacy and Health Sciences.

I formulated a complete nutritional supplement line, which includes over 25 cutting edge products designed to work with the Metabolic Diet and to maximize body composition, athletic performance and the beneficial effects of exercise. These formulations were done using the latest scientific and medical information, along with the knowledge and expertise I have accumulated in the last four decades. I have tried to use the best ingredients available regardless of costs to form products that are superior to any on the market today. These supplements, plus my latest book, *The Metabolic Diet* along with related books and ebooks **(www.MetabolicDiet.com),** form the nutritional backbone of some of my new international ventures.

I am now in the process of releasing new supplement formulations for my new international Signature Series of nutritional supplements and developing my two web sites, **www.MetabolicDiet.com** and **www.CoachSOS.com**. The goal of the new sites is to provide specific and detailed training, diet and nutritional supplement schedules for anyone including those who just want to lose some weight and/or bodyfat, to those who want to train for a specific activity or sport, including recreational sports, team sports, bodybuilding, Olympic events, and all the various other power and endurance sports.

My new book, The Anabolic Solution, written for both recreational and competitive bodybuilders, is an attempt on my part to present the ultimate cutting edge, training specific, diet and nutritional supplement guide geared to maximize muscle mass and minimize bodyfat. In fact my Anabolic Solution is so effective that it offers the only viable alternative to the dangerous use of muscle building drugs such as anabolic steroids, growth hormone, IGF-I, clenbuterol, thyroid, insulin, and countless others.

Photo Archive

My wild lifting days – picture taken in 1982, weighing around 195 lbs and getting ready to attack a 780 lb deadlift. At that bodyweight I had no neck to speak of. Neck measurement at that time was 19.5 inches.

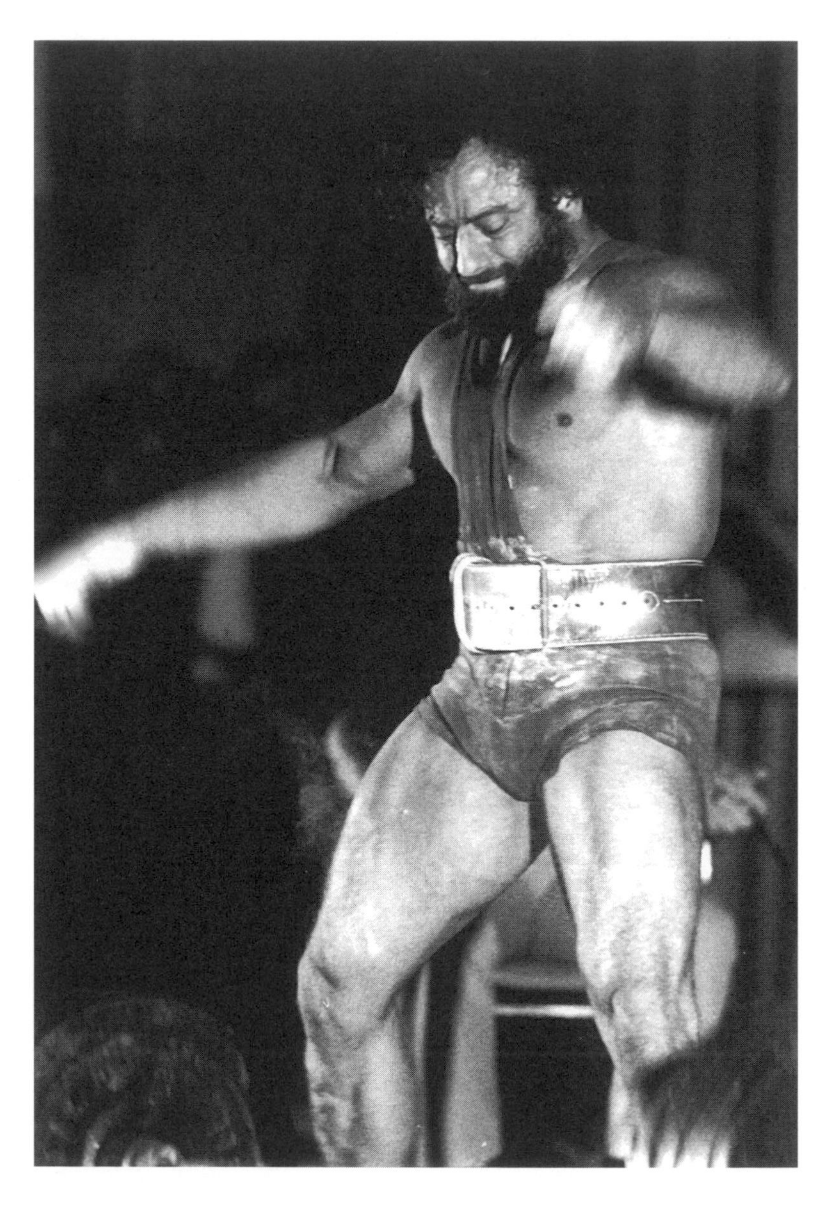

At the Beach in 1986 – weighing about 185 lbs at 7% bodyfat. And still with hair.

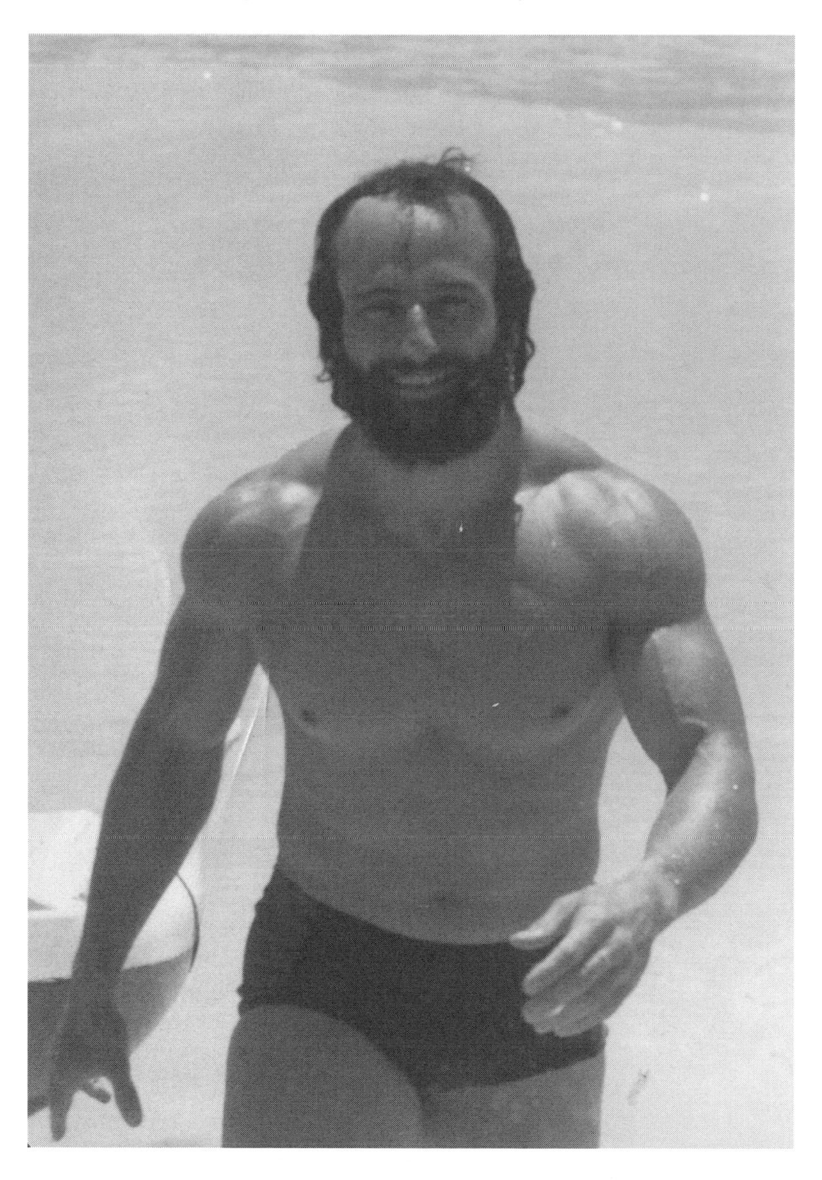

Eddie Robinson and Me in the summer of 1996, outside 10K Fitness – my gym in Cobourg, Ontario, Canada. Bodyweight was just over the 200 lb mark.

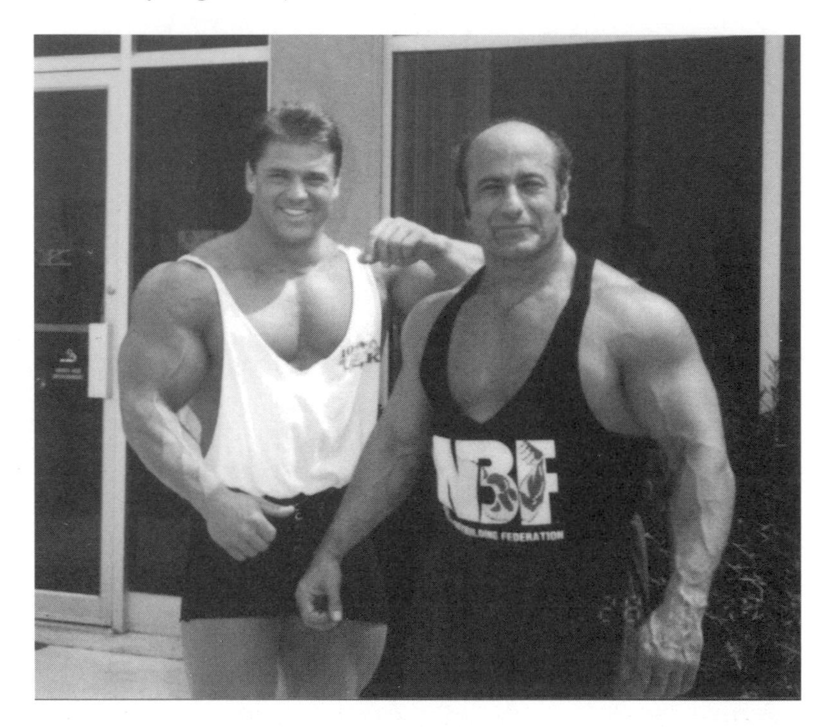

Tom Platz and I comparing pipes at my house in Cobourg in the Summer of 1996.

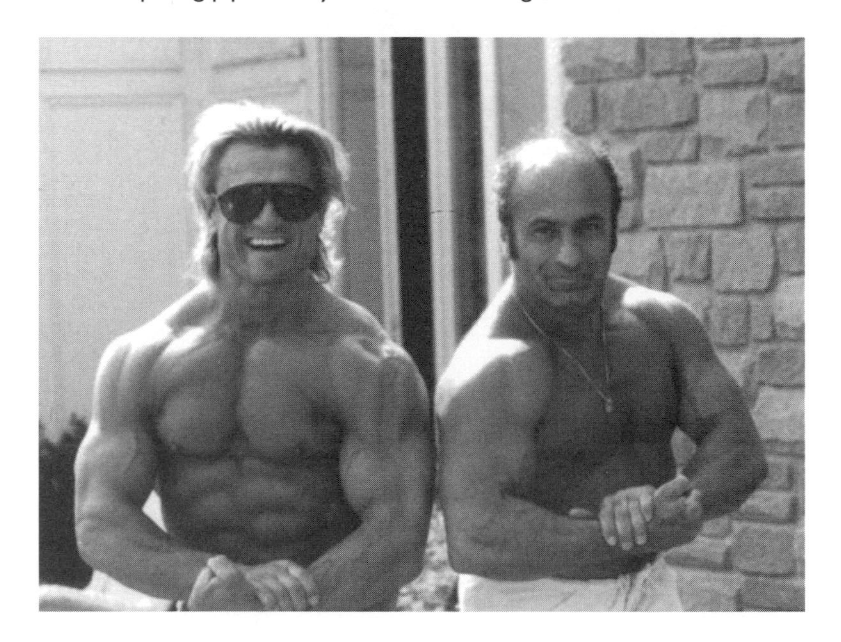

Picture taken in 1999 at the beach in Ecuador with some friends. Part of my South American trip as President of the Pan American Powerlifting Federation.

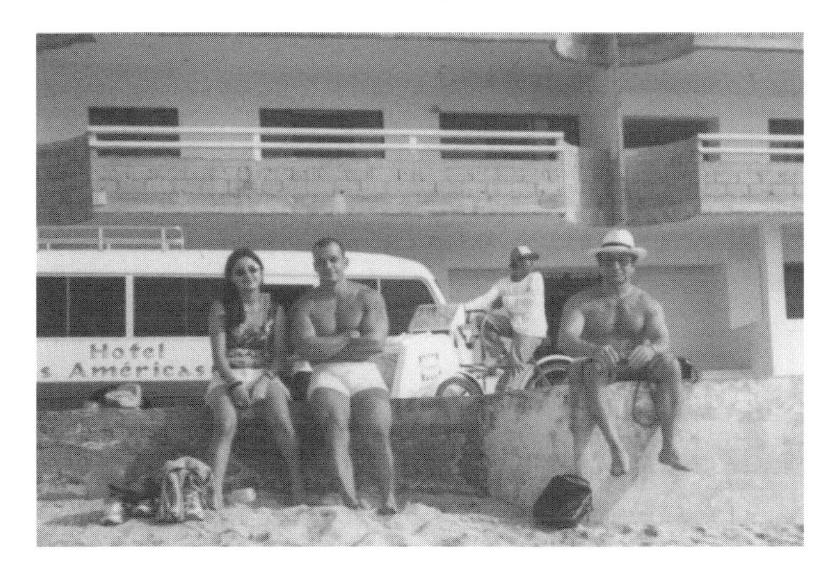

Formal picture taken in the fall of 2000.

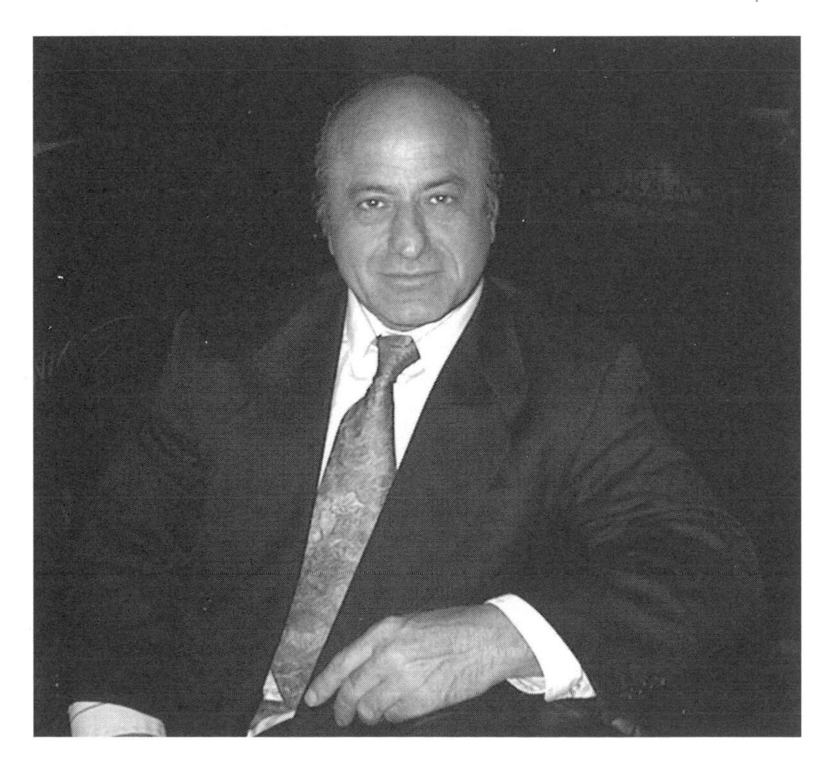

Preface

I meant The Anabolic Solution to be a simple guide for bodybuilders on how to best use the Anabolic/Metabolic Diet to maximize muscle mass and minimize bodyfat. But it has become much more.

First of all it is a simplified guide on how to use the Metabolic Diet and my targeted line of nutritional supplements in the different training phases. It's also a valuable source of information on nutrition and supplements and on macronutrient metabolism – how macronutrients are used and interconverted by the body. As well, it's an extension of my two major web sites, **www.MetabolicDiet.com** and **www.CoachSOS.com**. You will also soon be able to log on to **www.AnabolicSolution.com** where we will be both posting information as well as directing you to relevant sections in my other sites.

I have written this book to make is easy to understand and follow. But parts of this book are also quite technical. I felt it was important to present some of the more technical information so that you can understand how everything fits together and as such make more rational nutrition and training decisions, and make better progress.

So how should you use this book? It all depends on your level of knowledge and expertise. The best way for the uninitiated or less experienced bodybuilders, at least for the first reading, is to just read the instructional parts and leave the technical details for another reading or for referencing down the line.

Since the Metabolic Diet is the cornerstone of my Anabolic Solution, I thought I'd put in some of the basic and starting information for the Metabolic Diet right at the start. Thus the introduction will immediately detail everything you need to get an overview of how and why the diet works, and to get going on the diet ASAP. In fact I have overdone it in some ways in order to get certain points across, to the point where I maybe even repeat myself once or twice.

By doing it this way it gives you the kernel of information you need to get started ASAP or at least to get enthused enough to read anything else you need to know. Later chapters will have more details and explanations on how to best combine the Metabolic Diet with periodized training and the use of nutritional supplements. The more technical information can be read at leisure or on a need to know basis.

Whatever you read and in whatever sequence you read it, just remember that the basic principles behind the Anabolic Solution are easy to understand and follow. Also that the principles espoused in this book are based on solid scientific principles and research, and real world use.

Introduction

The Anabolic Solution

The Anabolic Solution is all about manipulating lean body mass and bodyfat. And it does this by affecting metabolic changes and altering the body's anabolic and the catabolic hormones and growth factors. But it's more than just the best natural way to reach your bodybuilding goals. By duplicating much of what people get from the use of ergogenic and body composition changing drugs the Anabolic Solution is a safe, effective, and natural alternative to the use of these drugs.

The "just say no" to drugs mantra adopted by so many in our society is an exercise in futility, especially in the bodybuilding, fitness and sporting world. What we need, instead of all the naysayers, is a viable alternatives to drug use. And that is just what we have in the Anabolic Solution.

Besides offering the best bodybuilding system in the world, and a viable alternative to drug use, the Anabolic Solution explains both the art and science behind the use of the Metabolic Diet and sophisticated nutritional supplements, explaining why and how they work and how they can best be used.

The Metabolic Diet is a revolutionary diet that uses macronutrient shuffling to accomplish its body composition magic. The effects of the Metabolic Diet are synergistically enhanced by the use of sophisticated, targeted nutritional supplements in various training phases.

In this book, we will show you when, where, why and how to use the Anabolic Solution to get results you never thought possible without the use of drugs.

Why Natural is Better

When you use drugs you are short-circuiting your body's normal processes. By providing hormones and other substance from outside the body, you shut down the internal mechanisms that would normally produce that substance. This is easier to understand if we use the analogy of a factory producing some goods. If we provide the goods that the factory would normally make, then there is no need for the factory to be operational. If the factory is shut down long enough then sometimes it's hard to get it up and running since we have to round up the workers and raw materials, and get everything working at peak efficiency again.

The same things happen to our internal factories when we provide outside hormones and drugs. Whatever processes are involved in making these compounds, or in doing the things that these compounds do, are thus no longer needed so they are essentially shut down. This can result in long term and sometimes a permanent imbalance in the body that can be harmful to your health.

An example would be the use of anabolic steroids in males. Their use shuts down all the hypothalamic, pituitary and testicular (evidenced by shrinking testicles) processes involved in the production of testosterone. After they are discontinued, in the time period during which the body is getting back to normal, most of the results and advantages of using drugs, are invariably lost. But it can even be worse than never having gone on the drugs since in some cases the systems never really return to normal.

On the other hand by maximizing the stimulation or activation of your internal factories, along the lines that they would naturally be stimulated in the first place, all you are doing are maximizing the input, the operation and the output of your own body, making it hum along at peak efficiency.

As well, by staying natural, we avoid the possible short and long-term consequences of drug use. These include short and long term changes in hormonal, metabolic and homeostatic processes and possible tissue and organ dysfunction. The long-term consequences of using some of the ergogenic and body composition changing drugs are yet to be determined but may well result in significant cardiovascular, hormonal, and carcinogenic (cancer producing and/or promoting) consequences.

We will have a bit more to say about all this in Chapter One where we describe the Metabolic Diet in some detail. Couple the effects of the Metabolic Diet with the use of effective nutritional supplements, and use these in specific ways in different phases of training and you have got a natural, safe and effective system for making progress and reaching your goals, without drugs.

Just keep in mind that by using drugs you force your body to adapt in ways that it's not meant to, and that the changes brought on by drug use may have significant short and long-term consequences. By using the Anabolic Solution your body is in control, and changes in ways that are compatible with short and long term health, with results that are comparable to those obtained with the use of drugs.

The Metabolic Diet

The cornerstone of the Anabolic Solution is the Metabolic Diet. So we will work on that first. While most books have you sift through a lot of introductory, basic and theoretical information before you get to the part you are really interested in. That is not the case here. We are going to tell you what you need to know in this introduction.

Metabolic Diet Set Point

The first thing I want you to understand about the Metabolic Diet is that it's a living, breathing entity, and not a static diet like all the rest. In other words it takes into account the differences in the ability to use carbohydrates and fats that exist in people, and allows them to individualize the diet to suit their own unique metabolism. As such, at the heart of the Metabolic Diet is the notion of your **Metabolic Diet Set Point**.

YOUR METABOLIC DIET SET POINT IS THE LOWEST LEVEL OF CARBS THAT YOU NEED TO FUNCTION OPTIMALLY, WHILE AT THE SAME TIME MAXIMIZING BODY COMPOSITION.

The fact that you can figure out the best level of carbs that suits your metabolism while at the same time maxing out your ability to increase muscle mass and decrease bodyfat, makes the Metabolic a "Holy Grail" of diets.

For some people, those that are efficient fat oxidizers and have little need for dietary carbohydrates, the Metabolic Diet Set Point will be less than 20 grams a day. For a small number of people, the Metabolic Diet Set Point may well be high enough that it ends up being a high carb diet. Most, however, fall somewhere in-between, usually between the 30 to 100 grams of dietary carbs per day. Almost as important as the amount of carbs is the timing of the carb intake.

When you have to increase the level of carbs in your diet it will take a while before you discover what your carb set point is (see Problem-Solving Guide). I have found that it takes people about two months on the average to find their ideal dietary carb level. Once you discover your Metabolic Diet Set Point, you can fix your diet at that level for several months while you work on changing your body composition.

The Metabolic Diet is based on three steps and principles that explain how it works and why it's the best diet for maximizing muscle mass and minimizing bodyfat.

1. In order to change your metabolism to burning fat as your primary fuel, you replace the carbs you are eating now with protein and fat, without changing the calorie level. The body adapts to the lack of carbs by priming up its fat burning machinery – increasing lipolysis and the oxidation of free fatty acids.

2. Once you are fat adapted (i.e. your body depends mainly on both dietary and bodyfat, not carbohydrates or muscle protein, to produce the energy it needs) you can cut calories by cutting the amount of fat in your diet.

   As the amount of fat in the diet naturally decreases, the body then uses bodyfat as its primary fuel.

3. Changing your metabolism to a fat burning one, and cycling from low carbs to a short phase of high carbs, allows you to naturally maximize muscle mass and minimize bodyfat. This is done by manipulating the major anabolic, anticatabolic, and fat burning hormones including testosterone, growth hormone, insulin, insulin-like growth factor I (IGF-I), cortisol, and thyroid.

The Three Priorities of the Metabolic Diet

1. Priority number one in the Metabolic Diet is switching your metabolism to burning fat as its primary fuel. This is done by limiting dietary carbohydrates and providing ample dietary fat. During this adaptation stage you do not really need to change your normal caloric intake. Simply substitute protein and fat for your former carbohydrate calories. An easy way to do this is to stick to mainly meat, chicken, fish, eggs, hard cheeses, salads (watch the carbs in the dressing, and no croutons) and whatever vegetables you want (except for the starchy vegetables like potatoes, carrots and peas). As far as what to drink, that is easy too. Water, diet drinks, coffee and tea (with cream and artificial sweetener only) are about it. That means no juices or any sugared drinks.

2. Once you are fat adapted, the next priority is to vary your calories to suit your goal. To increase muscle mass you increase your daily caloric intake by increasing fat and protein in your diet. It's usually a good idea to do a controlled weight gain first and then to drop that extra bodyfat while maintaining the most of the muscle you packed on while you gained weight.

3. The third priority is to refine your physique so that you are muscular and lean. To lose bodyfat while at the same time maintaining muscle mass, you slowly decrease your caloric intake and at the same time your fat intake. By providing less calories and dietary fat, your body will use its fat stores, not muscle, more and more to make up any energy deficits. In some circumstances, because of lower dietary fat levels, your diet may contain only moderate or even low levels of fat, mainly in the form of the essential and monosaturated fatty acids.

The Metabolic Diet's Four Practical Steps

1. Replace the carbs you're eating now with protein and fat – don't drop your calorie level right at the start.
2. For the first cycle, stick to the low carb phase for a full 12 days before beginning the high carb phase.
3. When you carb up, end carb loading the minute you start smoothing out.
4. Once you're fat adapted (usually after the first two weeks, change the calorie level depending on the training phase you're in, i.e. mass, strength or cutting phase.

The Metabolic Diet Works Because...

- ➔ Your body learns to burn fat instead of carbs.
- ➔ Your body continues to prefer fats as you drop calories, mainly in dietary fat and, depending on your dietary carb intake, some carbs. Always keeping protein high to spare muscle.
- ➔ As calories drop, bodyfat becomes the main fuel even if you lower dietary fat dramatically.

Also...

- ➲ Cycling from low carbs, high fat to high carbs and lower fat manipulates the anabolic and fat burning hormones and processes in the body to maintain or increase muscle mass while at the same time decreasing bodyfat.

Remember...

- ➲ You teach the body to burn mainly bodyfat in preference to carbs and protein.
- ➲ By shifting from a low carb diet on weekdays to a higher carb diet on weekends, you manipulate the muscle building and fat burning processes and hormones.

CHAPTER ONE

Dietary Carbs and Fat – Views Are Changing

I have advocated a lower carb diet for over three decades because I always felt that it was the best diet to maximize muscle mass and minimize bodyfat. I feel that each one of us has what I call a carbohydrate set point – the lowest level of carbs that you need to function optimally, while at the same time maximizing body composition. In most cases this level is quite low, at least relative to present thinking.

Both my earlier Anabolic Diet and now my more sophisticated Metabolic Diet and Anabolic Solution take the low carb equation to a level above all the other low carb diets, not only because the carb level is matched to each person individual genetic makeup, but also because it involves a macronutrient shift. This shift from low to higher carbs is meant to increase the anabolic effects of the diet by making use of the anabolic effects of insulin while at the same time limiting insulin's effects on fat metabolism.

The lower carb, phase shift diet that I developed (initially as the Anabolic Diet) and refined into the present Metabolic Diet, has caused some skepticism because of the low fat craze that has enthralled North Americans the past twenty years. But the winds of change have been sweeping over us recently and we are all starting to look at the low fat, high carbohydrate mantra with more skepticism and acceptance.

There are many reasons for this new acceptance of a higher fat, lower carbohydrate diet. For one, the last two decades, during which the low fat, high carb lifestyle was king, have seen an unprecedented rise in obesity, the exact opposite of what was supposed to happen.

We are also realizing that fats are not the villains they have been made up to be. The results of a study published in July, 2002, showed that the long term use of a low carb diet resulted in increased weight and fat loss, and a dramatic improvement in the lipid profile (decreased cholesterol, triglycerides and LDL, and increased HDL levels).[1]

As well, we are finding out that different kinds of fat can have varying effects, many beneficial (except for trans fatty acids – a type of fat found in margarine and many processed and fast foods) on serum lipids.[2] Even stearic acid, one of the major saturated fats in beef, which has been a target for low fat fanatics, has been shown in a recent study not to have any adverse effects on cholesterol levels.[3] While the oleic acid in beef has been shown to lower LDL cholesterol.

Recently there has been an increased emphasis on the importance of essential fatty acids and monosaturated fats (such as olive oil) to both our health and body composition. As well, we are seeing that high carb diets have adverse effects on serum lipids,[4] both the triglycerides and, partly because of the low fat part, cholesterol (unsaturated fats like olive oil are good for you and tend to elevate levels of HDL – the "good" cholesterol, and lower LDL levels – the "bad" cholesterol).

Effects on Body Composition

On top of all this, a number of reputable researchers have published studies that back up much of what I have been saying all along about the effects of low carb diets on body composition. The newest study to add credence to my views looked at body composition and hormonal response to a low carbohydrate diet.[5]

That is not to say that there hasn't been other research showing that a low carb diet results in a significant fat loss and an increased retention of muscle mass, either alone or in comparison to a high carb diet.

For example back in 1971 a group of researchers looked at the effects of three diets that had the same calorie and protein levels, but varying fat and carbohydrate levels.[6] They found that as the carbs in the diets went down, there was an increased weight and fat loss. In other words the men that were on the lower carb diets, lost the most weight and bodyfat.

In 1998 another study, this time involving obese teenagers, came up with similar results.[7] After 8 weeks on a low carb diet the teens not only lost significant amounts of weight and bodyfat, but they even managed to increase their lean body mass.

In the present study a six-week carbohydrate-restricted diet resulted in a favorable response in body composition (decreased fat mass and increased lean body mass) in normal-weight men. The results of this study indicate that a low carb diet mobilizes and burns up bodyfat more than a high carb diet, while at the same time preserving muscle mass. Magical words to almost everyone I know.

While this research backs up the first part of my dieting program, the second aspect, the macronutrient shift, has yet to be studied. This is about to change, however, as I am in the process of working with some top researchers on this aspect of the diet. Preliminary results are showing the advantages of this phase of the diet, and I will be releasing these results in future issues of Muscle Media.

Dietary Fat Is Not the Enemy

Even though views are beginning to change with many people it's still the same story. In fact you have heard it all before. Everybody from the American Medical Association to the media trendsetters to that so-called "expert" at your neighborhood gym has been saying the same thing for the last three decades. Fat is bad. Carbohydrates are good. If you want to get the body you have been working so hard for, you have got to focus on those carbohydrates and keep fat to an absolute minimum.

So you dedicate yourself to living by the percentages the "lowfat experts" give you. 55 percent carbs. No more than 15 percent fat. You load up on turkey and chicken. You separate the egg whites. You surgically remove all visible fat from any piece of meat. You always broil. Never fry.

But you have been living a lie.

Fact is, the high carbohydrate diet favored by so many bodybuilders can actually work against them. They bulk up on all those carbs and end up packing on a tremendous amount of bodyfat. Then, when it's time to cut, too much muscle ends up being left in the gym along with the bodyfat.

Strength levels and personal motivation drops. You can become irritable. Maybe even depressed. By the time that contest you have been working so hard for comes around, you often look no better than you did for the last contest. You may look worse.

And that diet. To say it's inconvenient and strict would be a drastic understatement. In a world where eating makes up a great part of our social life, the regimen of a high carb, low fat diet can quickly make you a social outcast.

Not that you cannot make progress toward your goals with a high carb diet. You can. Some. But you can also find yourself plateauing or even losing lean body mass. And if you try and get as lean as you can, you can suffer a dramatic loss in muscle mass. It's even worse if you are trying to get contest ready. As you count down toward contest time, panic can set in. You take drastic measures to compensate for the state you are in and end up losing weeks of training.

So, why are you torturing yourself? Especially when there is an alternative that can pack on muscle while keeping bodyfat at a minimum. It's called the Metabolic Diet and, while it flies in the face of what most bodybuilders have been led to believe, it could be the answer to your prayers.

The Metabolic Diet

Unlike the high carb diet that can work against the body's system of growth producing hormones, the Metabolic Diet maximizes the production and utilization of the Big 4 growth producers – testosterone, growth hormone, insulin-like growth factor I (IGF-I) and insulin – and does it naturally. It also shifts the body's metabolism from that of a sugar burning, fat producing machine to that of a fat burning machine. With the body packing on extra muscle and simultaneously burning both dietary and stored bodyfat, the bodybuilder finds himself twice blessed.

The Metabolic Diet stresses an initial high fat/high protein/low carbohydrate approach to nutrition. Many in the general public will dismiss it out of hand citing the popular beliefs that fat is a prime component in heart disease, cancer and obesity. Likewise, many bodybuilders have come to assume the dietary fat smoothes the bodybuilder out and blurs definition.

But they could not be more wrong. Dietary fat, when utilized properly as in the Metabolic Diet, can be the key to growth and success. And while some will see the Metabolic Diet as a new, revolutionary, even dangerous approach to nutrition its basics actually originated with the dawning of mankind.

The Primitive Diet

First let us clear up a widely held misconception that ancient man was a herbivore who turned his nose up at all meat in favor of the available plant life. Current vegetarians often claim that their diet is the most natural and ancient known to man in an effort to gain converts but it's simply not true.

In fact, archeological evidence shows that man's earliest tools were put to use, at least in part, in the dressing of meat. In many areas, the diet of primitive man was made up almost entirely of animal products. The continued affection for meat demonstrated by the monkeys and apes that are our primate cousins today is also testament to early man's dietary preference.

There is a good reason for all this. It's called survival. Meat is a far superior source of amino acids than plant life. It's also high in vitamins A, E and B complex. Vitamin B12, while plentiful in meat, is not found in vegetable products. Red meat is loaded with iron that is easily absorbed, unlike iron that is present in many plant sources. As well, red meats are excellent sources of potassium, zinc and magnesium.

Fat, whose benefits we will discuss throughout this book, is also readily available in meat and not in plants. Along with many other uses, including the fact that it's tasty and adds to the palatability of food, fat is necessary for proper breakdown and use of vitamins A, D, E and K in the body.

Meat is, indeed, one of the most nutritious substances on earth and it's been held in high esteem by civilizations throughout history. It's even played a big role in religious ceremony. In the early days of recorded history meat was offered to the prevailing Gods through "burnt offerings" and the Bible reports on feasts held in conjunction with these animal sacrifices.

So when we are talking about "natural" or "primitive" diets we are not talking about the eating habits of vegetarians. We are talking about meat eaters who came to understand early the importance of meat in the daily diet. Man's earliest diet probably consisted mainly of meat supplemented by periodic feedings of carbohydrates. It was only with the development of agriculture a mere 10,000 years ago that any large change was seen.

In the nearly 50 million years of man's existence before that, man was largely carnivorous and lived off animal flesh. At its crudest, this meat diet bears a strong resemblance to the Metabolic Diet we will be providing you with. All we have done is taken this primitive diet and brought it into the modern age making use of modern science to adapt it and perfect it for maximum health, fitness and development.

In response to this, some people will argue that the domesticated meats available today are fatter than the wild meats consumed by our ancestors and also fatter than the meat from wild animals today. While this is true, it's only a matter of degree. In the Metabolic Diet the quantity of fats is as important as the quality since we use the increased fat intake to shift our metabolism and thus make constructive use of the increased amount of polyunsaturated, monounsaturated and saturated fats without incurring any of the potential bad effects.

The point I want to make here is that meat is not inherently bad. Our ancestors ate meat to some degree for many thousands of years and we are genetically built to make maximum use of all it has to offer. On the other hand, we also have the capabilities to manage and use various kinds of plant food. After all, our evolutionary process has taken us through many dietary phases where both meat and plant foods were in our diet in various proportions in a continuum between the two extremes. The all meat diets to all plant diets.

If we look at the overall picture and take into account the various phases of man's evolution, the one lesson to take home when we discuss our ancestors' eating patterns is that because of varied eating patterns, man has had to undergo a diverse evolutionary process. As a result of this process we have the genetic ability to use fats, including stored bodyfat, as our main energy source, an ability that is not utilized fully by those of us on today's high carbohydrate diets.

The Establishment Will Not Like the Metabolic Diet

But do not expect the Metabolic Diet to be hailed widely by major food industries in our society. Go down the aisles of any supermarket today and all you will see on the shelves are various fancy ways to package carbohydrates. On the other hand, meat is simple. And while you can package it different ways, it's hard to disguise or to package for big profits. It would not be in the interest of the major food industries to support this diet. The bottom line rules.

A similar situation exists with the run of the mill vitamin and nutritional supplement industry. Most of the supplements they tout will be of little use here. That is because when you are on this diet you need supplements that do more than the cheap formulations (but not necessarily cheap in price), bottom line companies supply.

On the other hand there are supplements that will give you a big boost in achieving your goals. The ones that I will be suggesting are my own line of supplements that are high tech and specially designed for the needs of the bodybuilder dialed into the anabolic lifestyle. These supplements, which are way beyond the useless stuff that the bodybuilding and fitness supplement industry often fills their shelves with, will give you the edge in maximizing the anabolic and fat burning effects of exercise and the Metabolic Diet's benefits.

Most of today's nutrition experts who think that the quality of a diet should be measured in its high carb, low glycemic carb content, will not be pleased with this diet, either. After all it goes against many of their most sacred, but misguided, beliefs.

Also, the Metabolic Diet isn't as nitpicky as most diets out there and so it's easy to follow. You will be eating meat during the weekdays supplemented by a wide variety of other delicious foods. And when the weekend comes, virtually anything goes.
While you may have to give up that lasagna or ice cream during the week, you can have it during the "carb loading" portion of the diet that comes every weekend. Unlike both the high fat and the permanent low carb diets, you aren't forced to give up your favorite foods forever on the Metabolic Diet.

The History of the Metabolic Diet

Prior to 1990 most bodybuilders and power athletes followed a diet that was high in protein and complex carbs and low in fat practically all year round. The only thing that varied, except when they fell off the diet, was the calories – higher when they were trying to gain muscle mass and lower when they were cutting up. As such the staple power and muscle mass diet, especially among bodybuilders, consisted of a lot of high protein foods such as egg whites (the yolks, as nutritious as they are, were considered verboten as they contained some fat), broiled or baked skinless chicken, tuna packed with water and of course lots of oatmeal and rice.

All that has changed in the past decade. Ever since I introduced my Anabolic Diet to the bodybuilding community in the early 1990s, many power athletes, and especially bodybuilders, have gotten off the high carb/low fat bandwagon and gone on cycling lower carb, higher fat diets, maintaining the high protein edge. These bodybuilders, and their numbers are increasing daily, have found that they can get more massive and ripped on my diet than on the "traditional" bodybuilding diet. Although we will cover the basics and how-to below, my latest book, the Metabolic Diet (available on **www.MetabolicDiet.com**), outlines the diet in detail. There is also a lot of supportive material and a ton of articles, not to mention my complete Metabolic Diet Supplement line, on both of my main Internet sites, **www.MetabolicDiet.com** and **www.CoachSOS.com**.

The Metabolic Diet is not a new diet. Some of the principles have been in existence for several decades. For example, back in the 1960s a group of bodybuilders used a low carb diet with great success. However, it wasn't well refined at the time, nor did it feature the critical aspects of hormonal manipulation and stimulation I have added. But it concentrated on meat consumption with very few carbs and bodybuilders were pleased to find themselves maintaining maximum muscle with very little bodyfat.

In fact, the diet produced some huge men back in the 60's. They didn't have all the components of the diet perfected and didn't get the "super-ripped" look bodybuilders work for today but, nonetheless, the diet produced some big, big men. Unfortunately, the trendy diets stressing high complex carbs, high protein and low fat swept through the bodybuilding community so completely that these earlier experiments in a high fat approach were wiped out.
As often happens, the blinders went on to alternatives to the high carb movement and the higher fat, low carb diet was ignored by most people. I was the exception. I began working with the diet as an active powerlifter in the 1970's and used an earlier version of the Metabolic Diet on my way to winning the world championship in powerlifting in 1976 and the World Games in the sport in 1981.

Anabolic Steroids

At the time I was working on and using the Anabolic/Metabolic Diet, the world of professional sports began their campaign against anabolic steroids. Strict drug testing began in the world-class bodybuilding community and the cry went out for some natural alternative to steroids.

By that time steroids had assumed its place as a "wonder drug" among bodybuilders and other athletes. Physically, steroids had been shown to have a remarkable effect on muscle growth and strength. Psychologically, they provided users with an aggressive, contentious mindset very useful in competition and training. The fact that they swept through the bodybuilding and other sport communities where getting a competitive edge was so important to winning was not surprising.

Unfortunately, steroids were found to have some severe side effects. Moodiness and an unhealthy aggression toward others that could extend to violence (known as "road rage") were widely reported in sporting journals. Links to heart disease, liver cancer, kidney disease and sterility were also discovered. With the evidence mounting, there was little choice but to shut down their use in the international sporting arena.

Then in the early 1990s, because of some drug allegations against Vince McMahon and his sports federations, I was asked to handle the talent of both the World Wrestling Federation (WWF) and the World Bodybuilding Federation (WBF). Making sure that the athletes didn't use drugs wasn't enough however. We had to provide a viable alternative, especially for the professional bodybuilders that were in the WBF.

It was into this void that I stepped with my Anabolic Diet and the new approach to dieting I'd been working on. It wasn't an easy task. The World Bodybuilding Federation wanted their athletes to get clean but maintain muscle mass and stay cut up and in competition shape. This was a tall order.

Figure 1. The Hypothalamic-Pituitary-Testicular Axis (HPTA)

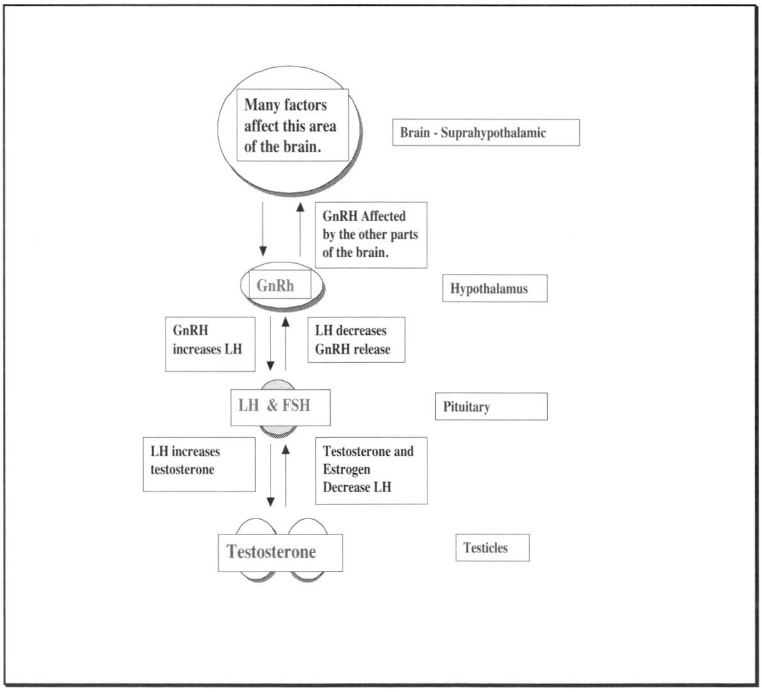

Abbreviations:

- GnRh – Gonadotropin Releasing Hormone
- LH – Luteinizing Hormone

One of the major problems was to get the hormonal systems of the bodybuilders back on track producing testosterone naturally. This was very difficult because steroids shut down the testosterone producing system in the body. The hypothalamic, pituitary, testicular axis (HPTA – see Figure 1), the axis that controls testosterone production, ceases to function and you may need to go to extreme measures to get your testicles working again. It often takes a long time to recover and, in some cases, a user may never recover and be doomed to treatment with artificial steroids or testosterone for the rest of his life.
Steroids can also make the athlete lazy. He will get growth with marginal training methods but find the road much tougher when he gets off steroids and has to do all the work himself. Metabolic diet or not, it may take him awhile to get back up to speed with proper training methods.

Then there is the diet itself. Like any diet, if you do not follow it you are not going to get results. Some bodybuilders who'd been cruising on steroids for a long time found it difficult to replace the ease of steroids with a diet that required some commitment.

Finally, some people chose to believe that a natural program could replace steroids (and the dozens of other drugs, such as growth hormone, IGF-I, insulin, thyroid hormone, diuretics, etc.) immediately and offer the exact same results. There is no way this can occur. Over a short time period, no diet is going to replace steroids. But over the long term, the Metabolic Diet, coupled with high tech nutritional supplements, has proven to be a very effective alternative to steroids providing the same kind of results without the "Russian Roulette" nature of steroid usage,

By 1990, I'd come out with my book "Beyond Anabolic Steroids" and begun to provide articles for a variety of fitness and bodybuilding publications on the subject. A few years later I started writing on my new diet system and in 1995 wrote the Anabolic Diet. The response to the Anabolic and the newer Metabolic Diet has been remarkable. In a world where steroids are a real gamble, both in terms of competition and health, the Anabolic and Metabolic Diets gave the bodybuilders who used it that natural edge they were looking for.

But I am no "Just Say No" crusader in this area. Hysteria is not my stock in trade. Anabolic steroids do have their place. In fact, I have been involved in research testing steroids for use in AIDS patients. They could play a role in maintaining body mass and strengthening the immune system in these patients thus allowing them to better resist the opportunistic diseases that are so deadly to them.

I also fully realize that steroids and other artificial means for growth and performance are still used widely in the athletic community. They give the athlete the edge he's looking for and, for many, they will gladly risk their health and the sanctions that can come from steroid use for the performance benefits they can bring.

It should be pointed out that the Metabolic Diet can be used in concert with steroids. You will get results. Indeed, you can do most anything with steroids and achieve some gains. But, though the Metabolic Diet will help you to some degree, your use of steroids will keep you from maximizing some of the endogenous anabolic hormones the diet seeks to stimulate, particularly endogenous testosterone.
Bottom line, the Metabolic Diet is really meant for the natural athlete who wants to be the best he can be naturally, but it works for anyone, with or without drug use. And, while it's much easier and convenient to stay on than the high carb diet, it will still require some dedication and the will to properly execute it. The key to success in the diet is to make sure you take your body through a "metabolic shift" where you will begin to use dietary fat and bodyfat instead of carbs and muscle protein as the main fuel for your body. To do this, you will have to follow the diet very closely, especially at the beginning.

The battle the drug-free athlete engages in is not an easy one. He must face up to drug-using and abusing competition and drug-based competitive standards in every contest. What the Metabolic Diet does is to give him the same kind of benefits the drug user obtains.

By introducing anabolic drugs or agents into his body, the drug user increases the circulating amount of anabolic hormones and other compounds, which in turn produces the desired anabolic effect of muscle growth. The Metabolic Diet does the same thing. Only instead of introducing the anabolic substances from an exogenous source outside the body, the diet stimulates the production of anabolic hormones IN THE BODY. It's LEGAL and it's SAFE.

And, best of all, it's a SURE THING. If you follow the diet, IT WON'T FAIL. It may sound bizarre. It may counter everything you have ever been led to believe about diets, fat and carbohydrates. BUT IT WORKS. It is a biochemical inevitability. YOU WILL get the combination of increased lean body mass with less bodyfat you are looking for if you follow the diet properly.

And you will get it naturally. Without the dangers of steroids.

Given the trials and tribulations most bodybuilders have experienced with their "diets", what more can you ask from a nutrition program?

Competing Diets

In the last 40 years I have seen a lot of accepted dietary 'truths' come and go. The most important thing I have learned in all this time is that you have to keep an open mind and be flexible enough to adjust your views according to the never-ending parade of new facts and information that comes on the scene.

The high carbohydrate, low fat, low to moderate protein diet is an outdated diet who's time has almost run out. Even though the attitude of those in the know towards these kinds of diets has changed, the new diet information has not reached the kind of critical mass it needs in order to become the logical successor to the diet crown.

So while I, and many others, believe that the Metabolic Diet is the most advanced, scientifically based diet plan on this planet, there is still a vocal majority that hasn't discovered the vital facts and as such still sticks to the high carb, low fat idioms.

However, I know that a paradigm shift will soon occur as the new dietary information hits the critical mass and becomes accepted by the majority of people as the best diet for those who exercise and want to increase their strength and muscle mass and decrease their bodyfat levels.

The Options

There are all kinds of diets out there. Low fat, high fat, low carb, high carb, low protein, high protein, hospital, vegetarian, limited food, wine lovers diet, and all the mixes and matches you could imagine. The more popular ones are the high carb, low fat diets, the low carb diets and the high protein diets (see Figure# – anticarbohydrate vs. antifat). All these diets have several subsections that treat the macronutrients differently but for our purposes we can lump them together under the broad categories.

Figure 2. – Anticarbohydrate vs. Antifat

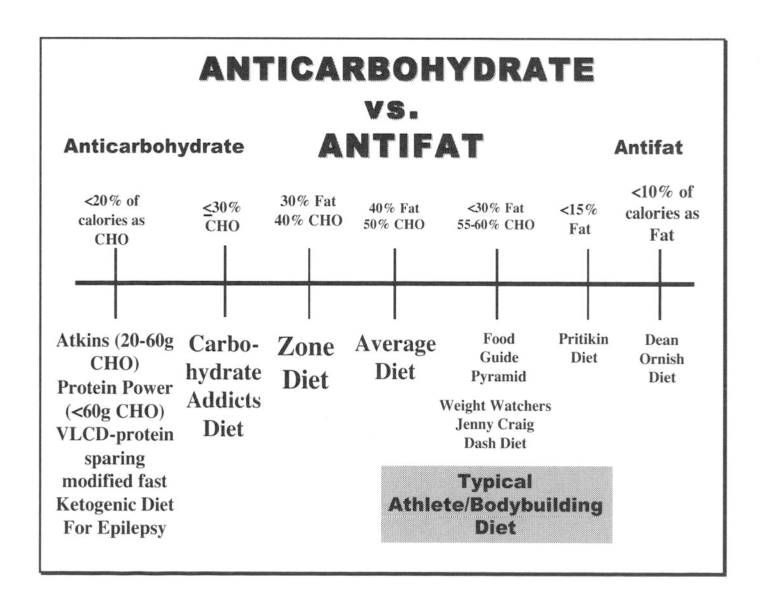

The High Carb Low Fat Diet

The high carb, low fat diet is the most popular diet on this planet. That is due in part to the fact that this diet is mostly plant based and thus readily available to people all around the world, especially those in third world countries. It also has been the subject of a lot of research and is espoused by the American Dietetic Association and other health professionals. The premises behind this diet is that by cutting down on fat you cut back on the one macronutrient that provides the most calories and as such you lose more bodyfat. Not only that but the weight of popular opinion is that fat is bad and lowering dietary fat makes for a healthy heart.

Unfortunately both premises are flawed. First of all by cutting down on dietary fat you actually burn less bodyfat and tend to lose more muscle. So by cutting back on calories you will lose weight but a lot of that will be muscle. The end result isn't pretty since to get in contest shape, or even to reduce your bodyfat to acceptable levels, you are going to lose a lot of that hard earned muscle.

There are also some health concerns regarding the high carb diets. Recent studies have shown that the high carb diet raises serum triglycerides and lowers HDL and as such can lead to an increase in cardiovascular disease. And if that is not enough, the low fat diets can be too low in the essential fatty acids and may result in a problem with the absorption of the fat soluble vitamins including vitamin A, D, E and K.

High Protein Diets

There are various kinds of high protein diets. Some are based on low fat and low carbs, and more along the ketogenic diets, such as the Atkins' Diet. Others are based on moderate carbs and fats, like the Zone Diet, or high to moderate carbs and low fat, and are just a variant of the high carb, low fat diets mentioned above.

In all cases the high protein levels are useful for those who exercise or are involved in sports. However, those that are low in fats and/or high in carbs run into the same problems as mentioned above with the high carb, low fat diets.

Low carbohydrate diets such as the Atkins' Diet and other strictly ketogenic diets are great for losing body weight and dealing with some health issues such as glucose resistance and diabetes. However, long-term strictly ketogenic diets tend to result in decreased muscle mass. That is because they do not allow alternating periods of lower and higher carb days. These alternating periods allow for favorable changes in the anabolic and fat burning hormones.

The Zone Diet is a good all round diet that stresses lower carb and fat levels and higher protein levels than is found in general diets. It's a good diet for losing weight while at the same time maintaining muscle mass. In fact, it's pretty close to the Moderate Carbohydrate Phase of the Metabolic Diet. Unfortunately, the Zone Diet suffers from the same fatal flaw as all the other diets out there.

None of them are up to snuff because they are all static diets based on fixed macronutrient content. The fact is that the one-diet-for-all approach just doesn't cut it genetically.

The Metabolic Diet on the other hand is a flexible living entity that is able to adjust to your needs, while at the same time finding the optimal carb level for maximum muscle mass and fat burning capability, and peak efficiency. By using the Metabolic Diet you can dial in your metabolism to the kind of diet that is best for you.

Diet Books

Most of the diet books on the market today are so similar that the same person could have written them. This includes books by physicians, PhD's and all the Jenny Craig/Susan Power types. They all offer variations of the diet high in complex carbs and fiber and low in fat. They also push exercise, lifestyle and behavior changes. Regrettably, none of these diets has much chance for success when the novelty has worn off and motivation wanes.

The reason they do not work is that they are basically all the same and usually depend on the personality of the writer rather than any real differences in the diets. Once a dieter has tried one of them they have tried them all, no matter how well they are disguised. None offer the novelty and biochemical advantages of the Metabolic Diet where you can lose bodyfat in even stubborn areas while maintaining or even improving muscle tone and body shape. Unlike the rest, the Metabolic Diet is not a fixed diet and is the first diet that can be adjusted to suit your metabolism.

You also have to remember that a lot of these books were written by people who had weight problems themselves and lost the weight through the use of personalized methods. Because of this, they are wildly evangelical in their praise and biased to flaws in their diets. There is very little, if any, science or research support for many of the claims they make.

CHAPTER TWO

The Metabolic Diet

The Metabolic Diet is the Holy Grail of diets in that it is the first scientifically based diet that can be adjusted to suit your individual and unique metabolism. It is the first diet that understands that each individual has a different genetic make-up and as such needs a personalized diet.

METABOLIC DIET

- Is scientifically based.
- Not a fixed diet like all the others.
- It's the first diet that can be adjusted to suit your metabolism.

Benefits Of The Metabolic Diet

More Muscle, Less Bodyfat, And It's All Natural

For more than 20 years the American public has been told to watch its fat intake or suffer the consequences. The national "fat hysteria" got so bad that back in 1989 the National Academy of Sciences advised everybody, regardless of the presence or absence of risk for coronary heart disease, to go on a restricted diet low in fat. The Lords of Lowfat loved this and the food industry proceeded to take advantage of the situation, as they always do, and come out with a whole new line of "lowfat" or "fat free" products, many of which were neither.

Why groups such as pre-menopausal women and children, who are largely immune to coronary heart disease, should go on such a restricted diet was not explained. Meanwhile, other complex, interlinking causes of coronary heart disease like lack of exercise, obesity, stress, genetics and caloric intake went largely ignored. Fat was the culprit. Any possibility that dietary fat could be utilized in the cause of good health and physical performance was conveniently dismissed.

As a result, people began eating those carbs. They began watching what they ate. Above all, they became aware of the fat they were eating and did their best to avoid it like a plague.

And, guess what? As a society we got fatter than ever. We are getting fatter all the time. The heart attack parade hasn't stopped. What's wrong with this picture?

Meanwhile, bodybuilders didn't seem to be getting the kind of growth they were looking for from all those carbs. Sure, they got big. But they also got fat. By contest time, they were most often right about where they'd been before they started the whole diet cycle. The siren song of steroids became ever more inviting.

But now, you have got an alternative. A healthy and effective one. It's called the Metabolic Diet and it's been striking telling blows against the Lords of Lowfat and getting bodybuilders the growth they want without all that added bodyfat. In this chapter we will outline the many benefits to be gained from the Metabolic Diet and begin to look at the reasons why it works. By its end, I do not think you will be too tempted to return to the old grind of that high carb diet.

Physical Benefits

Increasing Lean Body Mass WITHOUT Anabolic Steroids: This is one of the real big advantages of the Metabolic Diet. As described in the previous chapter, the diet does many of the same things hormonally that steroids do, only naturally inside the body and without the risks.

Decreasing Bodyfat Without Sacrificing Lean Mass: Unlike the high carb diet, when you gain weight on the Metabolic Diet much less of it is bodyfat and much more of is muscle. We have found that, far from what you have been led to believe, eating fat doesn't lead to getting fat. In fact, high dietary fat is instrumental in increasing lipolysis or the breakdown of fat and the resulting loss of bodyfat. We have also found that the bodybuilder will maintain more lean body mass during the cutting phase of a diet.

On the high carb diet, if you exercise correctly and do everything else right, you will find that when you lose weight about 60 percent of it is fat and 40 percent muscle. You may get down to your optimum weight and be ripped but you are much smaller than you could be. On the Metabolic Diet, we have found those percentages go way down to 90 percent fat and 10 percent muscle and that is a real boon for the bodybuilder who wants to maintain muscle as he cuts down. With the high fat diet you get down to the weight you want but find yourself maintaining a lot more lean body mass. You are bigger and stronger.

Take two athletes, one on the high carb diet and one on the Metabolic Diet, have them gain 10 pounds and you will find the one on the Metabolic Diet gaining the larger percentage of muscle. Likewise, when you lose weight the athlete on the Metabolic Diet will lose far less muscle than the athlete sold on high carbs. Which diet would you rather be on?

Feeling Stronger While Losing Bodyfat: This stands to reason. Strength is proportional to muscle mass. When you are on the high carb diet sacrificing lean mass to get cut, you are obviously going to feel weaker. Because the Metabolic Diet cycles in a carb loading phase every week to stimulate insulin production and trigger growth, you also do not find yourself getting into the psychological doldrums you get following one diet all the way through each week. There is a variety in your diet and this will aid you in being more energetic and committed than you'd be on the high carb diet.

Maximizing The Effects of Endogenous Anabolic Hormones: This diet maximizes the serum levels of testosterone, growth hormone and insulin to promote growth. It basically conditions your hormonal system to create an endogenous (natural) anabolic (growth producing) environment. It tries to maximize the effect of these 3 anabolic hormones 24 hours because, contrary to popular belief, you do not only get stronger and form muscle just after a workout but, if you do it right, during a workout as well.

This is one of the most remarkable effects of the Metabolic Diet and it doesn't come easy. Many hormones are reactive to others. For instance, as insulin goes up growth hormone may decrease. If insulin decreases, growth hormone will increase. The two substances generally do not work together but they can. If you can increase both substances, you will get a better anabolic effect than with an increase in one substance alone.

Later we will provide some supplements that you can use with the Metabolic Diet that will help in increasing insulin, testosterone, growth hormone and IGF-I as needed. For example, **Exersol**, which is made up of three formulas targeted for use before, during and immediately after your workouts. This is especially important because of the decrease in serum testosterone and growth hormone that can occur during and after a workout.

At the cellular level in the body, you need the anabolic hormones elevated so they will drive amino acids into the cell for protein formation. That is how you get growth. The Metabolic Diet, the weekly cycling it incorporates and supplements will work to do this before, during and after your workout.

Increase In Strength: People on the Metabolic Diet often find that, as they are losing weight and bodyfat, strength increases. Most bodybuilders find this amazing. They know that when they lose weight they are also losing muscle and strength. But with the Metabolic Diet they're losing far less muscle and that, in combination with the fact their body is working in an anabolic environment, makes them stronger. They cannot believe it as they watch the fat melt away while their strength increases at the same time.

Decrease In Catabolic Activity In The Body: The Metabolic Diet results in lower levels of cortisol, a hormone secreted by the adrenal glands that breaks down muscle (catabolism) and uses it for energy. The supplements we will be adding to the diet will also decrease muscle breakdown during and after the workout while increasing insulin and growth hormone levels at critical times to promote an anabolic effect. Put simply, you will be breaking down less muscle while adding more.

PHYSICAL BENEFITS OF THE METABOLIC DIET

- Increasing Lean Body Mass Without Steroids
- Decreasing Bodyfat Without Sacrificing Lean Mass
- Maximizing The Effects Of Endogenous Anabolic Hormones
- Increasing Strength While Losing Bodyfat
- Decreasing Catabolic Activity In The Body
- Avoiding The Health Problems Of The High Carbohydrate Diet
- Staying In Shape Year Round Instead Of Peaking Once Or Twice
- Improving Contest-to-Contest And Year-to-Year/No Plateaus
- Endurance Increases

Avoiding General Health Problems Associated With The High Carbohydrate Diet: Carbohydrates will increase insulin levels and thus produce an anabolic (muscle building) effect when used properly. In the Metabolic Diet, we use a carbohydrate loading phase on the weekends to do just that. But when insulin is chronically high or yo-yos up and down due to a diet consistently high in carbs, it becomes a lipogenic (fat producing) hormone and begins to lay down fat on the body and plenty of it. That is why it must be controlled. You will note that on the Metabolic Diet the individual will increase carbohydrate consumption on the weekend only to the point when he begins to lay down fat. Then its back to the high fat diet before any damage is done.

This is why you tend to lay down so much more fat on a high carb diet. With insulin uncontrolled, you lay down fat indiscriminately. The chronic elevation of insulin also tends to deposit that fat in the thighs and other fat-plagued areas of the body causing the cellulite buildup that drives women especially crazy.

The increase in plaque buildup in the arteries that leads to heart attacks also appears to be a symptom of the chronically high carb diet. If you stay away from the simple sugars and junk food you can limit the damage, of course. It would be hard to severely criticize someone who eats a lot of vegetables, salads and potatoes.

Still, all those carbs will lead to fat buildup unless you regulate it as we do in this diet. Carbs are only increased to the point that they will have a beneficial effect on lean body mass. By spiking insulin production through carb loading on the weekends we can speed the movement of nutrients through the bloodstream and into muscle. Amino acids are driven into muscle cells where they can form the building blocks for protein and ultimate muscle growth. But before the insulin levels have been elevated too long and fat begins to be laid down in bulk, the carbohydrates are cut off and insulin brought under control.

Staying In Shape Year Round Instead Of Peaking Once Or Twice A Year: The Metabolic Diet allows you to stay in shape year round. It's not a diet where you bulk up and then cut bodyfat and the process becomes so painful and difficult that you cannot maintain the diet. As such, it's not one of those low-fat diets where you struggle mentally and physically all through the year and cannot help but go on and off it out of sheer exhaustion and frustration.

The Metabolic Diet is a lifestyle. One that you can keep up year round. It's very comfortable because it's natural. It punctuates high fat periods with regular carb sessions in much the same manner as our ancient ancestors' diet.

You also do not give up anything on this diet. You can have that meat and cheese on the weekdays and on the weekends load up with your favorite carbs. It's not torture like most other bodybuilder diets. You want to party and have a beer on the weekends? Go ahead. All foods are available, albeit at the right time of the week, on this diet.

Meanwhile, if used properly, this diet will allow you to keep your fat somewhere around the 10 percent level consistently and cut to a 4-5 percent as needed while maintaining lean body mass. There will not be those marathon cutting phases and you will find yourself getting into competition shape very quickly.

And, if you responsibly follow the diet and stay with it, each time you go through the cycle or complete your pre-contest phase you should come in heavier and at least as cut as you were at the end of your last cycle. Instead of plateauing as so many bodybuilders do, you will improve contest to contest and year to year.

Performance and Endurance Increases: We have also found that for many athletes endurance actually increases on the high fat diet. Again, this runs counter to popular belief that exercise endurance is related to the amount of carbohydrate stored in the muscle and that a low carb diet decreases performance.

In the high carb/low fat diet, the athlete begins training and as the glucose in the blood is used, liver glycogen is mobilized to maintain blood glucose while at the same time the glycogen or carbohydrate stores in the muscle are also used for energy. At the same time there is an increase in fatty acid oxidation and glucose formation from gluconeogenic precursors, mostly mobilized from muscle. Basically as exercise continues your body depends more and more on burning fat and muscle for fuel. Unfortunately, when you are on the high carb diet, your body isn't as efficient at burning fat and, unless some carbs are constantly supplied, you end up burning more protein (muscle) and less fat than you should.

Once you have shifted over on the high fat diet, though, your body is primed to use fat for energy.[8] In fact it uses up less of the stored glycogen in the liver and muscle and depends more on fat for its energy source. The glycogen is preserved and used when it's really needed rather than being wasted on lower level activity where fat is an effective energy substitute.

Fat becomes almost like sugar to the body and it will favor utilizing fat stores over muscle and liver glycogen stores for energy. In this way, less fat is stored by the body and more of it is used. The body is much less likely to make fat and more likely to burn it off.

And it gets even better if you exercise. That is because when you are fat adapted muscle fibers undergo a shift of the energy substrate from carbohydrates and protein (read muscle breakdown) to fats, and use glycogen even more economically during physical exercise. A higher percentage of lean body mass is the result.

While I have been espousing the benefits of my Anabolic/Metabolic Diets for increased athletic performance and endurance for over three decades, it's only in the past ten years, or so that many of my views and theories have been substantiated by research. While more studies are needed I will give you a brief synopsis of what the literature shows so far.

Several studies have found that animals, rats and dogs in particular, adapted to a high fat diet have increased endurance capacities[9,10] and, unlike what happens on a high carb diet, and do not have a decrease in endurance capacity even after recovery from a previous exhausting work bout.[11] The latter condition seems to be due to the increased storage and utilization of intramuscular triglycerides (fatty acids), while the former is due to the increased use of free fatty acids as fuel and to glycogen sparing.[12]

A similar tendency to increased endurance has been found in fat adapted humans,[13,14] although some studies (in both animals[15] and humans[16]) have not shown any improvement in exercise performance or endurance. The problem with most of the studies that did not show any performance enhancement secondary to fat adaptation is that in people on a constant high fat, low carbohydrate diet, muscle glycogen content is compromised and even though there is less reliance on glycogen, this lower glycogen content likely is a factor in limiting performance.[17]

While some studies have shown that endurance exercise is optimized by following a Metabolic Diet suggested macronutrient shuffle (carb loading after adaptation to a high fat diet),[18] others have not.[19] More studies are needed to examine the issues involved. Especially needed are studies that examine the effects on exercise intensity, endurance and perceived exertion when a long-term fully fat adapted athlete carb loads on a cyclical basis, as occurs in the Metabolic Diet.[20] More studies are also needed to determine the effects of fat loading on exercise performance.[21]

Maximizing The Effects of Endogenous Anabolic Hormones: This diet maximizes the serum levels of testosterone (even in women[22]), growth hormone and insulin (the Big 3) to help firm up and shape your body as you shed fat. If you are exercising, you will be surprised at how quickly you will be able to sculpt the body you want as these hormones work together.

This is one of the most remarkable effects of the Metabolic Diet and it doesn't come easy. Many hormones are reactive to others. For instance, as insulin goes up, growth hormone may decrease. If insulin decreases, growth hormone may increase. The two substances generally do not work together, but they can. If you can increase both substances, you will get better results shaping your body and keeping it firm than with an increase in one hormone alone.

Later we will provide some supplements that you can use with the Metabolic Diet that will help in increasing insulin sensitivity, testosterone, growth hormone and IGF-1 as needed. Some of you will be very serious about your goals and may be seeking to take the advanced path a bodybuilder normally takes. Others will just be interested in keeping the body firm and shapely. Your approach to supplements and exercise will be largely determined by how far you want to go in remaking your body.

Whatever your goals, you will find the Metabolic Diet an effective tool in taking the weight off, keeping it off and making your body look it's best.

Decreases In Catabolic Activity In The Body: By "catabolic" we mean forces that break down muscle and use it for energy. When existing muscle is broken down, your body will lose its tone and may become flabby. The Metabolic Diet, accompanied by proper exercise actually results in the body producing lower levels of cortisol, a hormone secreted by the adrenal glands that leads to catabolism. By lessening catabolism we insure that the body retains important muscle mass and tone while you lose weight.

It has been shown that the carb-loading phase of the diet results in decreased cortisol levels. In one experiment the hormonal effects of muscle carbohydrate loading manipulations followed by a carb poor diet were studied.[23] Carb loading provided decreased levels of cortisol not only during the carb-loading phase but also in the following carb-poor time period.

The Metabolic Advantage

At this point, a little biochemistry lesson may be in order so you can get a better idea of why the Metabolic Diet is superior to the competition. Adenosine triphosphate (ATP) is the source of energy for all metabolic activity in the human body. In order to get the energy the body needs for muscle contraction, breathing, brain cell function and virtually all other activities, ATP must be generated. People have gotten the idea that you must have the glycogen and the glucose that comes from carbohydrates for the body to produce and replenish ATP and survive.

What people do not understand is that the body can produce glucose without taking in carbs (gluconeogenesis) and that protein and fat can be used to provide energy and replenish ATP. It is a misconception that you must have dietary carbs to function. This is likely only true in some cases where a person may be genetically challenged as far as utilizing fats efficiently. And even in these cases it's unlikely that there will be a need for the extremely high levels of dietary carbs now being called for by various groups and agencies.

When carbohydrates make up the bulk of your diet, you basically burn the glucose (and other sugars which, like glucose, enter the glycolytic pathway) from the carbs as energy. Glucose enters the bloodstream and it's either used for immediate energy or stored as glycogen in the liver and muscles (remember our discussion of insulin earlier?). The glucose not stored as glycogen is made into triglycerides (bodyfat). When needed for energy, the stored glycogen is converted back to glucose and used up directly by cells or transported through the bloodstream to other body cells for conversion and use as energy.

When fat and protein make up a greater part of your diet, your body no longer relies on those large amounts of glycogen or glucose for energy. A good part of your energy comes from the use of free fatty acids in your diet or from the breakdown and oxidation of bodyfat. As we discussed, some of the energy will come from gluconeogenesis, the formation of glucose mainly from glycerol and amino acids. Instead of burning all the stored glycogen or glucose for energy, the body burns free fatty acids or triglycerides (the storage form of the free fatty acids) and the glucose that it makes.

Basically, a diet high in fat activates the lipolytic (fat burning) enzymes in your body and decreases the activity of the lipogenic (fat producing) enzymes. Dietary free fatty acids and triglycerides become the body's main energy source. The triglycerides are broken down to free fatty acids and some of the fatty acids are metabolized to ketones, which in turn can be used for energy by body cells. The use of ketones for energy is especially important to the brain that can only use glucose and ketones for energy. In short, the free fatty acids and ketones take the place of glucose and the triglycerides act like glycogen.

When carbs are the main form of energy to the body, the body produces insulin to process it and store it. This is all well and good but, as we discussed above, one of the problems with insulin is that it activates the lipogenic (fat producing) enzymes on the body and decreases the activity of the lipolytic (fat burning) enzymes. What this leads to is an increased storing of bodyfat and a decrease in the amount of stored fat that will be burned.

The exact opposite occurs on the higher fat/lower carb diet. After undergoing the "metabolic shift" from being a carb-burning machine to a fat-burner, lipogenesis (the production and laying down of fat on the body) decreases, and lipolysis (the burning of both dietary and bodyfat for energy) increases. You are burning fat as your primary fuel, and instead of using glycogen or breaking down precious protein, you will burn off the fat on your body for energy as needed.

This can have a big effect on overall bodyfat, and research documents the fact that while on a higher fat lower carb diet, weight loss is due to the almost exclusive loss of bodyfat.[24] In one study of ideal-weight human subjects, it was found that higher fat diets were accompanied by a very strong lipolytic (fat-burning) effect.[25] In another study focusing on obese subjects, it was found that, when offered high-carb/relatively low-fat diets or lower carb/relatively higher fat diets, the subjects on the lower carb diets lost significantly more fat.[26] Though prevailing wisdom would predict that the higher fat diet would simply make people fatter, they actually lost more weight on a high fat diet.

It may sound crazy, but that is the way the body works. Contrary to what most people believe, fat oxidation is regulated primarily by carbohydrate intake rather than by fat intake.[27] Once you have adapted to a higher fat/lower carb diet, fat doesn't beget fat. Despite what you have been told, a properly designed diet higher I fat and lower in carbs doesn't put fat on. It takes fat off.

Similar results have occurred in animal studies.[28,29] Meanwhile, I have seen the positive effects of a higher-fat diet time and time again in my own practice. The fat melts away. At the same time, as a bonus, body tone can be improved markedly thanks to the "protein protecting" nature of the diet.

Protecting Protein

One important by-product of the "metabolic shift" that takes place when you move from a high carb to a good, higher fat/lower carb diet is that fat protects protein in the body. When you are utilizing carbs as your main source of energy, the body tends to save its bodyfat and will preferentially take muscle protein, break it down and form glucose from it to burn as energy when the immediate energy stores are exhausted. This is why on a high-carb diet a significant amount of muscle catabolism can take place.

Exercise should play a role in any diet. Every doctor or fitness expert will tell you that. If you want to come anywhere close to getting the kind of weight loss you want and shaping up your body, exercise is a necessity. Unfortunately, with the high-carb/low-fat diet, once you have exhausted carb based primary and secondary energy stores you are going to start burning some muscle for fuel when you are working out.

The fact is that anytime you are exercising and the body needs energy it will break down what it needs, including muscle, to supply that energy. One of the ways athletes fight this is to sip glucose drinks during a workout. The body will not need to break down muscle as much for energy because it has an outside source of energy constantly coming in. The problem here is that with the constant glucose ingestion you get chronically elevated levels of insulin and a decrease in the oxidation of bodyfat. Instead of losing fat by exercising you are actually preserving it.

Fat works in the same way as glucose when you are on the Metabolic Diet. It protects the muscle by serving as an alternative, more available source of energy and it does this without having to take in more calories since the body has learned to oxidize bodyfat to provide that needed energy. So now when you exercise you do not need to take in carbs to spare your muscles. Your body will burn up your excess bodyfat to provide the energy it needs to exercise at the same time sparing muscle protein.

On the high-carb diet you may find yourself in a gym, happily working away, but you will be sacrificing muscle in the effort. If you look around you will find examples of people who seem to be at the gym all the time, working on the treadmill or step machines and doing some weight training, but they just do not look the way they should.

They may be slender, but their bodies lack tone and they are stringy or shapeless. With all the work they are doing they should be looking like one of the covers of the magazines they have got in front of them while they walk the treadmill but they are actually burning off muscle and sacrificing tone. You can bet they are not on a higher fat/lower carb diet.

The Metabolic Diet works against this tendency. Some muscle will be burned, but available fat will serve as an alternative to muscle as an energy source so a minimal amount will be lost.

What we are concerned with here is "catabolism" or the breakdown of muscle tissue. Again, I know it may sound strange, but although most people think that exercise only creates muscle it also breaks it down. Research upholds that the Metabolic Diet could well also be called the "Anti-Catabolic Diet." Along with enabling the body's hormonal system to better burn fat it decreases the amount of muscle that could be lost during a workout or just during day to day activities, by protecting muscle protein. This is very important to someone wanting to shape his or her body for maximum attractiveness and fitness.

Research has shown that the ketone bodies (beta-hydroxybuterate and acetoacetate) burned for energy in a higher fat/low-carb diet, actually decrease protein catabolism.[30] A study done on laboratory rats also showed that a combined treatment with insulin, testosterone and a high fat/high protein diet led to decreased loss of muscle protein caused by the catabolic hormone corticosterone.[31] Another showed higher protein gains and lower fat gains for rats on a high-fat diet.[32] The implications for similarly decreased catabolism in humans with the higher fat/lower carb diet are obvious.

In my own practice, I have also noticed that bodyfat seems to be more mobile when the Metabolic Diet is being used. As discussed above, when you begin to lose weight you often have a very hard time losing it in problem areas like the thighs, buttocks and stomach. Weight seems much more evenly lost throughout the body on this diet. Problem areas are much more easily attacked.

I have worked with many patients who get skinny from the waist up when they diet. The stored fat in the buttock, inner thigh and lower abdomen areas refuse to budge. No diet has ever successfully slimmed these areas. But with the Metabolic Diet they lost fat evenly throughout these areas. Much of the cellulite that has bothered these people throughout their lives disappears and this encourages them to take their weight loss and maintenance efforts further.

Fat distribution also seems more evened out with the Metabolic Diet. What fat remains on the body seems to be distributed more equally on the frame. You just do not have those pockets of fat that plague people. Fat is distributed in a more pleasing ratio across the body making any bodyshaping efforts on your part that much easier.

METABOLIC BENEFITS OF THE METABOLIC DIET

- Burning Fat Instead Of Glucose Promotes Lipolysis (Fat Breakdown)
- Burning Fat Instead Of Glucose Decreases Lipogenesis (Fat Production)
- Without Dietary Fat, The Body Stores Fat In Excess
- Muscle Protein And Body Tone Are Protected
- Bodyfat Is More Mobile And Pleasingly Distributed – Decreases cellulite.

CHAPTER THREE

Why It Works

The Metabolic Diet Works because it changes some of the basic metabolism in your body so it becomes a fat burning machine. Cellular metabolic flux (as we will illustrate) is dramatically altered when we change the dietary macronutrient content. Some pathways become more active than others and some processes dominate in the production of energy.

In all cases, the body will adapt to the macronutrient content of any diet as long as the diet provides certain essential nutrients.

ADAPTATION

- The body will adapt to the macronutrient content of the diet, no matter how extreme.
- Only stipulation is that the diet must provide certain essential macronutrients and micronutrients.

First of all it's important to realize that there are no essential sugars or carbohydrates. Also the reasons given for why we need carbohydrates are faulty. For example one of the main reasons is that the brain depends on them to function properly. In fact lactate is the preferred substrate for neurons and these brain cells can also metabolize ketones effectively. As well, other cells in the central nervous system cater to the main brain cells and supply them with energy derived from other nutrients. For example it has been shown that astrocytes shuttle nutrients to neurons.[33,34]

THERE ARE NO ESSENTIAL SUGARS OR CARBOHYDRATES

- There are essential and conditionally essential amino acids and essential fatty acids.
- But no essential carbs because like the non-essential amino acids and fats, the body can produce glucose and carbohydrates endogenously.

So Why Do We Need Carbohydrates? Most Common Argument is that they're Necessary for the Brain. **Not So!**

- Brain can metabolize lactate and ketones as well.
- Lactate (and other nutrients) also shuttle from astrocytes to neurons.
- Also, glucose can be produced as needed.

Glucose can be produced as needed by a process called gluconeogenesis. In this process other nutrients, including amino acids and glycerol (the backbone that makes up much of our bodyfat) can be converted to glucose or used directly as energy.

Although somewhat complicated, the Figure below shows how the body produces glucose internally from other substances including the amino acids, glycerol (source can be from the breakdown of bodyfat or from the diet), lactate, and pyruvate.

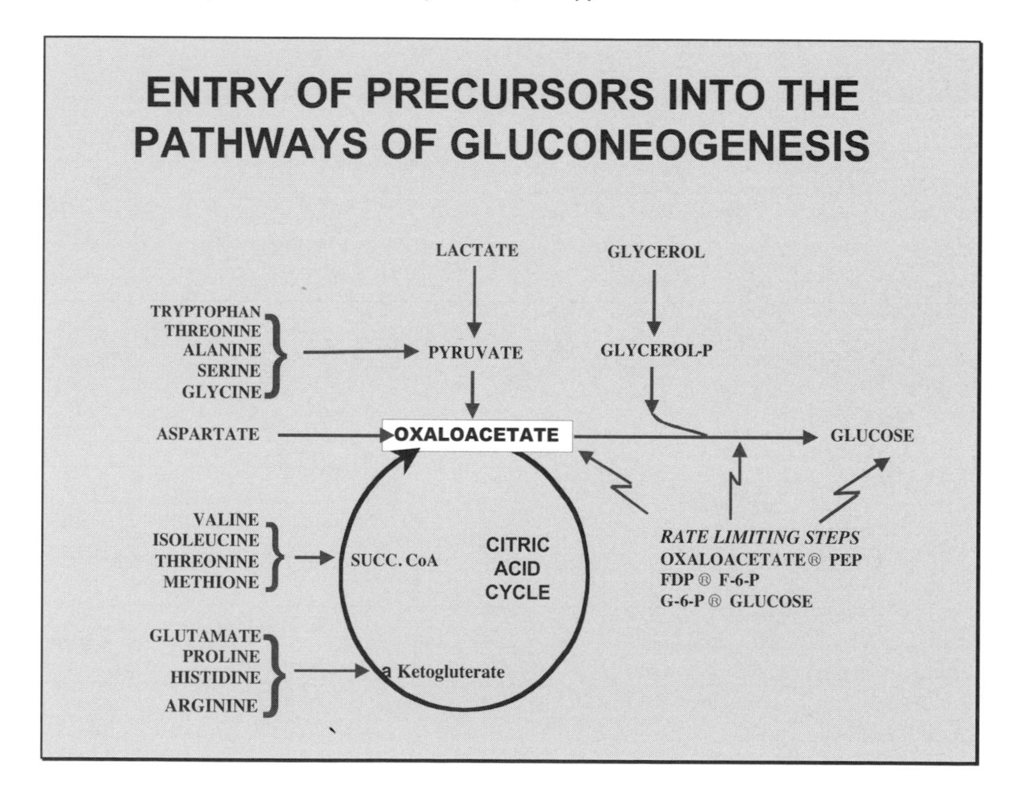

Because there are common pathways for the metabolism of all three macronutrients, variations in the macronutrient content results in adaptations that will allow the efficient production of compounds and substrates for energy production and body maintenance.

COMMON PATHWAYS FOR MACRONUTRIENT METABOLISM

- Regardless of the macronutrient mix the end results and the final pathways are the same.
- Interconversion of macronutrients, usually at some energy cost (conversion of protein to fats), and with some exceptions (inability to produce glucose from free fatty acids – although you can, to a limited extent, with triglycerides and bodyfat), is ubiquitous.

These next two diagrams shows how glucose, free fatty acids, glycerol and amino acids are broken down to provide energy.

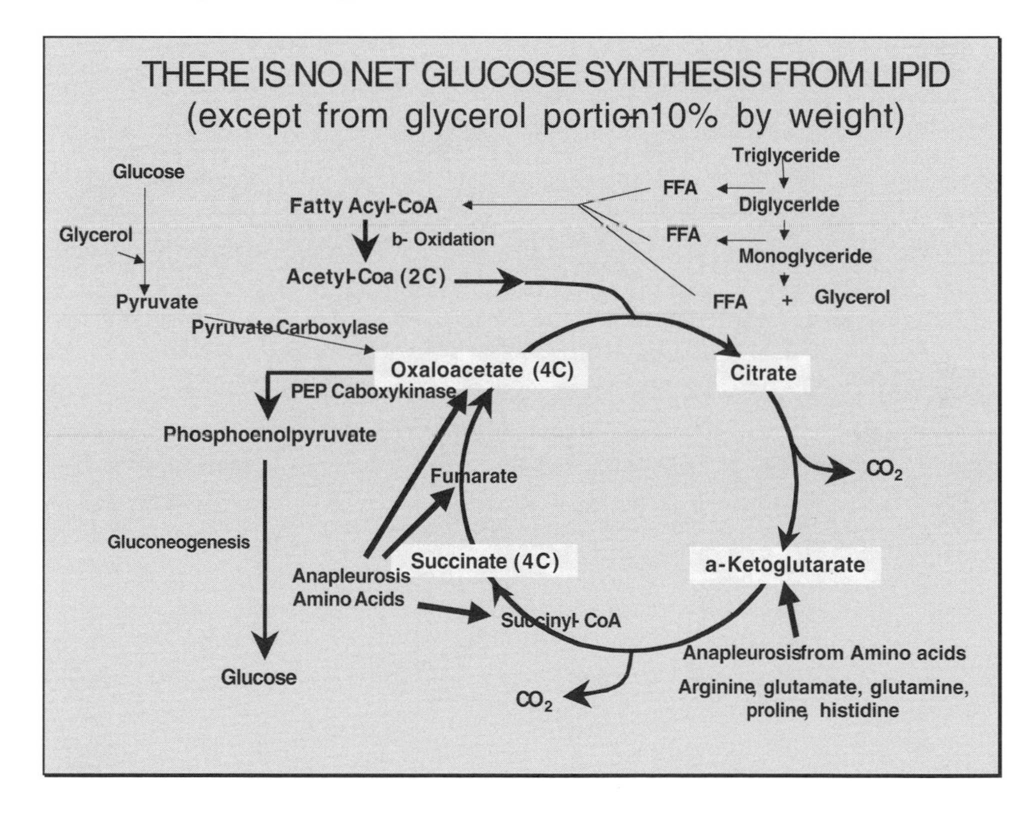

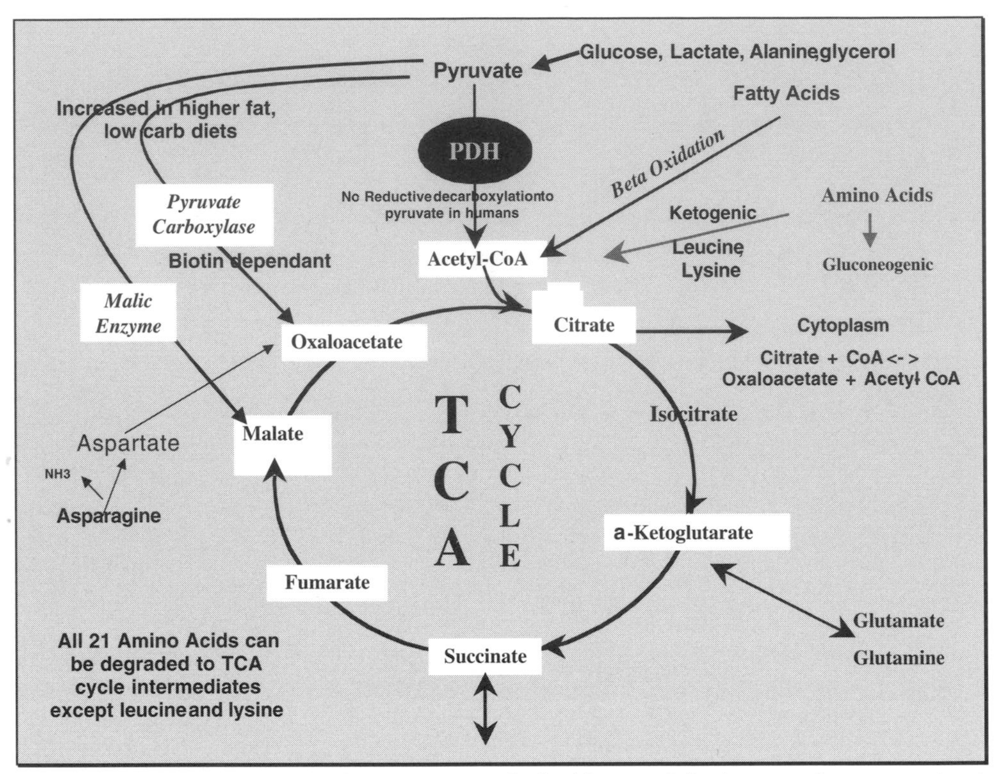

The Metabolic Diet controls the major muscle building and fat burning hormones in the body to maximize muscle mass and minimize bodyfat. These hormones include testosterone, growth hormone, IGF-I, insulin, thyroid, and cortisol.

REGULATING LIPOLYTIC ACTIVITY Major hormones are:

- Catecholamines (epinephrine and norepinephrine)
- Insulin
- Glucagon (more in forming ketones)
- Growth Hormone
- Testosterone

The Metabolic Diet also increases the activity of hormone sensitive lipase (HSL), the enzyme that breaks down bodyfat (lipolysis).

Hormone Sensitive Lipase (HSL) Adipose tissue lipolysis is stimulated through a cascade of cellular signals, resulting in activation of HSL.

But controlling the formation (lipogenesis) and breakdown (lipolysis) of bodyfat isn't enough. We have to insure that the fat that is broken down is also used up by the body for energy (beta oxidation or fat oxidation) rather than used simply to reform bodyfat.

Beta Oxidation of Fatty Acids

- The Other Side of the Fat Equation
- Lipolysis is of no use if the fatty acids are not used up.
- A paradox.

Not only does the Metabolic Diet increase fat breakdown but it also increases the use of fat as fuel for the body's energy needs. It does this in part by increasing GH, IGF-I and testosterone levels and partly by controlling the increase and sensitivity of insulin

The Metabolic Diet also increases the anabolic and anticatabolic hormones in the body including growth hormone, IGF-I and testosterone (including an increase in the androgen receptor and binding).

Increase In Both Lipolysis and Fat Oxidation

- Must have both otherwise may be counter productive.
- For example, a recent study shows that ephedrine like compounds increases lipolysis but decreases fat oxidation so that overall effect may be an increase in bodyfat.

  Mora-Rodriguez R, Hodgkinson BJ, Byerley LO, Coyle EF. Effects of beta-adrenergic receptor stimulation and blockade on substrate metabolism during submaximal exercise. Am J Physiol Endocrinol Metab. 2001 May;280(5):E752-60.

Other Hormones and Compounds

While we have dealt with the effects of the Metabolic Diet on several hormones and functions, there is much more to the story of how the Metabolic Diet works.

Some of this has to do with the way the Metabolic Diet manipulates other less know but very important hormones and compounds in the body, including leptin, ghrelin, and the hypothalamic hormones neuropeptide Y, agouti gene-related protein (AGRP), proopiomelanocortin [giving rise to the active α-melanocyte-stimulating hormone (α-MSH) peptide], and cocaine and amphetamine-regulated transcript.

Leptin is produced mainly in fat cells, although both endocrine and neuroendocrine tissues also express it, and has effects on almost every system in the body. It acts primarily through central pathways suppressing appetite and increasing the metabolic rate. It also seems to have significant endocrine and neuroendocrine effects (such as it's effects on the pituitary, thyroid, adrenal, and gonadal axes). As well it has some peripheral effects, particularly it's effects on increasing insulin sensitivity, and on the gastrointestinal and immune systems.

Leptin levels are regulated, among other things, by overall fat mass and by higher calorie and carb intake. Cut back on food and your leptin levels drop. This tells the body, among other things, that you need to find food (hunger increases) conserver energy (metabolic rate decreases) and preserve energy stores (especially bodyfat). In other words your body is preparing for the worst scenario, starvation. Increase your food intake and leptin levels promptly rise doing a lot of good things like decreasing hunger and increasing metabolic rate, but some bad things like increasing bodyfat.

The interesting thing about leptin, at least from our viewpoint, is that it reacts much faster than any significant changes in body composition. That is leptin will increase or decrease before there are any changes in bodyfat levels, which it helps to bring about. That means that there is usually a time gap between increases and decreases in leptin and the following changes in bodyfat.

And we make use of this phenomenon in the Metabolic Diet on the weekend when we increase both our calorie and carb intake – something I suggest later on when talking about the Cutting Phase. It's in this phase that leptin levels are affected because of the decreased calorie intake. Increasing carbs and calories jumps the leptin levels back up for the weekend carb phase, with all the benefits of leptin but without the adverse effects on bodyfat.

Ghrelin is a recently discovered peptide that is primarily produced by the stomach. It stimulates GH secretion but it also stimulates feeding and increases the formation of fat cells, at least in rats. In one recent study, low carb, high fat intake reduced ghrelin levels, and as such decreased appetite and fat formation. This is one of the ways that the body limits fat formation on a high fat diet. Again on the weekend, by increasing calories and carbs, we can make use of ghrelin quick effects of increasing appetite and GH levels, but avoid the slower effects of ghrelin on increasing fat cell mass.

It's beyond the scope of this book to cover any of the hormones and other factors we manipulate via either the Metabolic Diet and the use of various supplements. Suffice it to say that many of these were taken into account when I wrote the Metabolic Diet and formulated my line of advanced supplements.

How It Works

The Metabolic Diet – Fat Burning and Muscle Sparing

The Metabolic Diet works because it:

- Switches your metabolism to burn fat instead of carbs as its primary fuel.
- Maintains the fat burning as you drop calories so that the energy needed is obtained mainly from bodyfat not glycogen or muscle protein.
- Spares protein and maintains or allows you to build muscle mass.

The first step in the Metabolic Diet is switching your metabolism to burning fat as its primary fuel. This is done by limiting dietary carbohydrates and providing ample dietary fat. During this adaptation stage you do not really need to change your normal caloric intake. Simply substitute protein and fat for your former carbohydrate calories.

The second step, once you are fat adapted, is to vary your calories to suit your goal.

To increase muscle mass you increase your daily caloric intake by increasing fat and protein in your diet.

To lose bodyfat while at the same time maintaining muscle mass, you slowly decrease your caloric intake and at the same time your fat intake. By providing less calories and dietary fat, your body will use its fat stores, not muscle, more and more to make up any energy deficits. In some circumstances, because of lower dietary fat levels, your diet may contain only moderate or even low levels of fat, mainly in the form of the essential and monosaturated fatty acids.

The Metabolic Diet Works Because...

1. Learn to burn fat instead of carbs.
2. Body continues to prefer fats as you drop calories, mainly in dietary fat and some carbs. Always keeping protein high to spare muscle.
3. As calories drop, bodyfat becomes the main fuel even if you lower dietary fat dramatically.

Also... Cycling from low carbs, high fat to high carbs and lower fat manipulates the anabolic and fat burning hormones and processes in the body to maintain or increase muscle mass while at the same time decreasing bodyfat.

Remember...1. You teach the body to burn mainly bodyfat in preference to carbs and protein.

2. By shifting from a low carb diet on weekdays to a higher carb diet on weekends, you manipulate the muscle building and fat burning processes and hormones.

CHAPTER FOUR

The Metabolic Diet Plan

In this section, we will learn how the Metabolic Diet can be used to maximize strength and lean body mass, while in later chapters we will cover the details on how to use the diet in the various training phases. But first, although we covered how and why the Metabolic Diet works in the previous section, let me clear up a few misconceptions about the diet some people may have.

Insulin

First, let us make it perfectly clear that, unlike other diets that espouse a constant low carb intake and consider it as such, insulin is not the enemy. We are not mounting a campaign against it. In fact, it's only a problem when it's chronically high or yo-yo's such as it does on a carbohydrate-based diet.

INSULIN

Has a persistent and dramatic effects on decreasing lipolyis. The effects of insulin persist even when insulin levels return to baseline values.

In fact in the Metabolic Diet we make use of the anabolic effects of insulin while at the same time avoiding it's bad effects on bodyfat and insulin sensitivity.

Unchecked, insulin adversely effects bodyfat by decreasing the breakdown and increasing the accumulation of bodyfat. What you want to do with insulin, and what this diet focuses on, is to increase it at the appropriate time and place so it works to add muscle mass and maximize it's anabolic potential by, among other things, increasing the flow of amino acids into muscle cells.

INSULIN MUST BE CONTROLLED

- Beneficial effects of insulin on protein synthesis and muscle metabolism.
- Beneficial effects of insulin on glycogen supercompensation.
- Counter productive effects of decreased lipolysis and increased lipogenesis.

What we do not want is fat built up at the same time. That is why insulin secretion is controlled and limited. Instead of the chronically elevated insulin levels of the high-carb diet, the Metabolic Diet carefully manages insulin during the dieter's week so you get it's anabolic benefits without packing on all that unwanted fat.

Controlling the Effects of Insulin

- Only allowing controlled increases in insulin for the desired effects on protein synthesis.
- Attenuating the effects of insulin on lipolysis and lipogenesis.
- Accomplished by pulses of insulin and controlled insulin increase at variable times on weekends.
- Increasing GH (and testosterone) at the same time as insulin. For example prior, during and after training.

Another plus of the Metabolic Diet is that there is a decreased effect of insulin on fat metabolism even during the carb-up phase.

Effects of Insulin on Fat Metabolism

After the phase shift on the Metabolic Diet there is a decreased effects of insulin on fat metabolism EVEN DURING THE CARB-UP PHASE.

Insulin also works its anabolic magic hand in hand with testosterone and growth hormone (GH). GH is very important because of its positive effects on increasing protein synthesis and decreasing muscle breakdown. During the weekdays when you will be on the higher fat/higher protein/lower carb portion of the diet, insulin levels stay fairly steady and do not fluctuate wildly, and growth hormone secretion increases. Along with stimulating a great environment for body shaping, GH also induces cells to use fat instead of sugar for energy thus increasing the burning off of bodyfat and limiting its production.

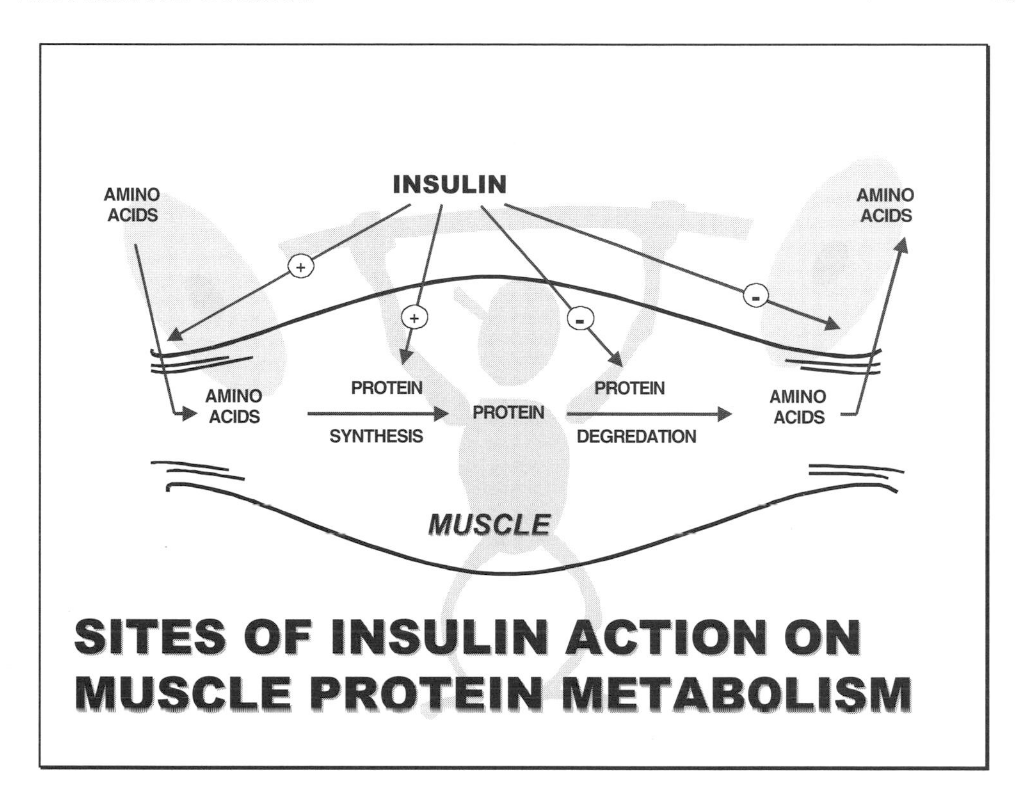

Growth hormone acts almost like a "starvation" hormone. When your body's in trouble or when you are threatened or in a dangerous situation, GH kicks in to mobilize stores of energy in the body to deal with stress and increased energy needs. GH levels also increase under the stress of exercise.

Usually insulin works to decrease the secretion of GH, but it appears that the body sees the great increase in carbs and insulin during the weekend portion of the Metabolic Diet as a stressful situation, much like exercise, and GH can actually increase with insulin. In this way, we potentially can get the positive effects of increased growth hormone both during the week and on at least part of the weekends.

Testosterone, Growth Hormone and Insulin-Like Growth Factor I (IGF-I)

METABOLIC DIET INCREASES GROWTH HORMONE, IGF-I AND TESTOSTERONE Increased GH and IGF-I secondary to decreased carb intake and amino acid effects.

Increased testosterone due to higher fat, higher protein and lower carb intake.

Testosterone, also critical to increasing muscle mass and strength, responds well to the Metabolic Diet. Preliminary research in this area has found testosterone is positively linked to dietary fat. In one study, pre-menopausal women placed on low-fat diets experienced decreased levels of both non-protein bound estradiol and testosterone (although postmenopausal women didn't experience the same deficiency).[35] In another promising study, animals fed diets high in cholesterol or fish oil experienced increased testosterone production over those fed a low cholesterol diet containing linseed oil.[36]

BIOAVAILABLE TESTOSTERONE Increased by diets high in fat and protein.

- Decreased in Vegan diets (as is IGF-I)
- Decreased in diets high in carbs.
- Even decreased if soy protein substituted for meat protein.

(Habito RC, Montalto J, Leslie E, Ball MJ. Effects of replacing meat with soyabean in the diet on sex hormone concentrations in healthy adult males. Br J Nutr 2000 Oct;84(4):557-63.)

A recent study showed that in older men the consumption of a meat-containing diet (like we recommend on the Metabolic Diet) contributed to greater gains in fat-free mass and skeletal muscle mass with resistance training than did a lacto-ovo vegetarian diet.[37]

Overall it has been my experience that there is an acute anabolic effect on muscle when a short-term lower carb diet is alternated with carb loading. Cellular hydration is maximized by the water and carb loading intracellularly, and insulin sensitivity is increased leading to an intense anabolic stimulus. Constant fluctuations make for an anabolic effect unparalleled by any other diet. This anabolic effect allows you to tone and shape your body as you lose weight.

Along with increasing the anabolic process in the body, it's also important to insure that the muscles you have developed aren't broken down. To do this you want to maximize the anabolic hormones such as testosterone and GH, and minimize the production and effects of catabolic hormones, the most critical of which is cortisol (cortisol also promotes fat storage). Much of this is done naturally through the Metabolic Diet. Since bodyfat stimulates cortisol production,[38] less cortisol is secreted, as bodyfat is lost.

ANABOLIC ACTION OF THE METABOLIC DIET Increases in bioavailable testosterone and in the androgen receptor.

- Increases in GH, IGF-I and IGFBP-3 and in tissue levels of IGF-I isoforms.
- Decreased cortisol levels.
- In concert with controlled insulin increases.

Psychological Control

Along with the hormonal control, you will also find the Metabolic Diet providing for psychological control. The wide mood swings and irritability you can get on a carbohydrate-based diet can also increase cortisone. In fact, psychological stress can be a prime component in its production.

The Metabolic Diet, in part by controlling insulin, can put a stop to the mood swings and irritability that plague the carb diets. It also minimizes the hunger, frustration and social stress created by other diets. Let us face it. Any diet can be difficult. It involves changing lifestyles and any change can be stressful. But the flexibility, convenience and simplicity of the Metabolic Diet go a long way toward getting rid of the stress that normally accompanies a diet.

The Importance Of Exercise

If you want to experience the maximum benefits from following the Metabolic Diet, you will need to exercise. Though it would be great to live in a world where you could go on a diet, spend the day in the living room couch and gain all the muscle and lose all the bodyfat and weight you want, this just isn't possible. And of course that is what this book is all about.

The Complete Picture

If you are going to give the Metabolic Diet your maximum effort, you will also need to get your training and nutritional supplements in gear. The diet itself -through the "metabolic shift" of changing the body over to a fat-burning machine instead of a carbohydrate-burning, fat-producing one – will melt away the bodyfat and give you the basics for creating a fit, attractive body. Exercise will give you a leg up on increasing muscle mass and decreasing bodyfat, while providing for good cardiovascular health and protection from heart disease.

Supplements will give you that extra edge to help get the maximum anabolic and fat loss effects out of the diet and training.

These three tools used together – the Metabolic Diet, a solid exercise program and a savvy approach to nutritional supplements – provide a "cannot miss" scenario for success. And to think it all occurs without the starvation and insanity that comes with the carb-based diets.

Getting Started

Before going on the Metabolic Diet you should get a complete physical from your doctor. You should also have some blood workup including complete a blood count, cholesterol levels (total, LDL, and HDL), TSH (a test for thyroid function), fasting blood sugar, serum uric acid, serum potassium, liver function array and BUN. Your doctor may want to go beyond this but he will let you know if you should have more done.

Dietary Fat

Your Cholesterol

As far as the cholesterol issue, because you are burning fat for energy, much of the cholesterol and saturated fats that could cause a problem are used up in the process. Studies have even shown that along with increasing the utilization of fat as an energy source and providing for weight loss, the Metabolic Diet can even reduce serum cholesterol.[39]

In fact the results of a study published in July, 2002, showed that the long term use of a low carb diet resulted in increased weight and fat loss, and a dramatic improvement in the lipid profile (decreased cholesterol, triglycerides and LDL [the bad cholesterol], and increased HDL [the good cholesterol] levels).[40]

In my patients, I have consistently found a reduction in serum cholesterol and an improvement in the cholesterol and triglycerides profile on patients who are on the Metabolic Diet and are losing or have lost weight.

A typical example is one patient who has been on the diet for two years. The table below outlines the changes in his lipid profile before he started the diet and after being on the diet for two years. During this time he has lost over thirty pounds while increasing his muscle mass, and presently weighs a muscular fit 200 lbs.

Table of Lipid Profile

	Nov-96	Normal Range	Nov-98	Normal Range	Comments
Total Cholesterol	236	160-240	220	175-260	Total Cholesterol Is Down
HDL	22	31-59	64	32-60	Good Cholesterol Is Up
LDL	191	90-171	141	104-179	Bad Cholesterol Is Down
Cholesterol/HDL	10.7	<5	3.4	<5	Total Cholesterol To HDL Is Down
LDL / HDL	8.7	1.52-5.52	2.21	1.73-5.59	Ratio of LDL To HDL Is Down
Triglycerides	123	10-150	72	10-150	Triglycerides Are Down

As you can see his lipid profile improved dramatically while on the higher fat/lower carb diet. His lipid profile taken two years ago would have put him in the high-risk category for coronary artery disease while the recent lipid profile puts him in the very low risk category in all the parameters presently used to assess this risk.

In this case, the patient was not all that careful in the type of fats he ate and did not take any oil supplements. He relied heavily on red meat. While some improvement would be expected from the weight loss and exercise, it's obvious that being on the Metabolic Diet didn't adversely affect his lipid profile.

On the other hand, it never hurts to keep track on your cholesterol level whenever you change diets and even more so if you have or have a tendency toward a cholesterol problem. Cholesterol levels are largely determined by individual metabolism and body chemistry, and genetics play a strong role. If you have had cholesterol problems in your family there is a good chance you may have them, too. And if you have a chronic problem with cholesterol you need to talk to your doctor about how this may be affected by the Metabolic Diet, and what you can do to limit any adverse affects. Frequent monitoring of your lipid status will let you know where you stand and if changes need to be made.

There are a number of adjustments you can make to the Metabolic Diet to control your cholesterol intake if needed. Marine oils, flaxseed oil, olive oil and other nutritional supplements will help. Meat restriction may also be necessary. But, again, this is something you need to work with your physician on. If the Metabolic Diet seems like the answer to you, you will have to put your heads together to devise a plan where you can benefit from the weight loss and toning advantages the diet provides while keeping cholesterol in check.

Also remember that the Metabolic Diet is as much a moderate to low fat diet as it is a high fat diet. It all depends on where you are at as far as the diet itself.

For example if your serum LDL and/or HDL levels are adversely affected by the diet at the beginning when you are adapting to burning fat as your main fuel, or when you are bulking up and taking in more fat, then the problem may correct itself as you modify the carb level to suit your metabolism or when you are in the process of decreasing your bodyfat such as when you go into a definition or cutting phase.

The solution to cholesterol levels that are worse on the high fat part of the diet is actually quite simple and is inherent in the way that I set up the Metabolic Diet. Keep in mind that the higher fat levels used initially in the Metabolic Diet are to help bring about the transition from carbs to fats as the main fuel for the body. Once this transition occurs fats are not as important as they once were.

In fact if you do follow a high fat diet to go through the initial fat adaptation or to bulk up, you must then lower the dietary fat levels as you shift gears to burn off that unwanted bodyfat. To do that you usually have to gradually drop your daily calorie intake, which means dropping your dietary fat intake since you obviously cannot decrease carb intake much as it's already low, and you have to keep protein levels high to maintain muscle mass. Thus you have to lower your dietary fat intake progressively until you reach your goal. As such, the Metabolic Diet moves from a high fat diet to a moderate and even a low fat diet depending on how low you drop your daily calorie intake.

I have found that once fat adapted, lowering dietary fat, as long as carbs are kept low, doesn't change the use of fat as the body's primary fuel. The body simply goes from using dietary fat to using endogenous fat as the preferred fuel. And that is one of the primary goals of the Metabolic Diet.

So if you are having cholesterol problems, the solution is obvious. You have to decrease your intake of saturated fats as much as possible and make up any calories that you lack with foods high in polyunsaturated/monosaturated fats (making liberal use of flax and olive oil), and high protein, lower saturated fat foods (for example steaks are OK but you have to take off all visible fat. Cutting back on egg yolk consumption, keeping the egg whites, is also a good idea).

Keeping Track

Along with getting the physical and blood work we also urge you to weigh yourself and get a bodyfat analysis before you begin the diet. Scale weight loss is important but so are inches. You should understand that there are times when, for a variety of reasons, you might not be losing much scale weight but you are subtracting that unsightly bodyfat. It will help keep your enthusiasm high in these moments if you know that progress is being made in other areas and your body is toning up. I have devised the Metabolic Index™ to help you keep track of your progress. By plugging in your weight, height and bodyfat level, you will get a good idea of whether or not you are losing bodyfat regardless of the changes in body weight.

In addition to keeping track of the Metabolic Index, you might also want to keep track of your body measurements. Especially important are your waist, hips, upper thigh, chest and upper arm. These measurements will give you an idea of how your body is responding to the diet and where you are losing weight the fastest. It will also give you an idea of where your problem areas may be and where you may have to concentrate exercise to get the body you want.

Secondly, measurements will be helpful for motivation when you are retaining fluid or not losing weight for some other reason and will complement the Metabolic Index. If you see those waist and hip measurements going down, despite the lack of weight loss, it will show you, along with the changes you will see in the Metabolic Index, that you are making progress.

Finally, you should review the use of any medications you may be on. If you are on diuretics, you may want to use them only as needed due to the higher fat/lower carb diet's ability to help you shed water.

Most Type I and Type 2 diabetics will usually have to adjust their insulin or oral diabetic agents, perhaps decreasing them during the low carb portion of the diet, and going back to their normal dosages on weekends.

You should check your glucose levels at various stages of the diet until you become familiar with the effect of the diet on blood glucose. It's important to check with your doctor and keep checking as you continue the diet and lose weight so that you are aware of your status and can make changes where needed.

The Diet – Where to Start

Although you can start the Metabolic Diet from two very different starting points I suggest that those who want to maximize strength and muscle mass and minimize bodyfat take the stricter, less complicated route. The original strict approach will allow you to most efficiently find your unique optimal dietary carb level.

The strict, low carb phase can last anywhere from two to several weeks and allows you to determine if you are an efficient fat user and as such can do quite nicely without too many carbs. If that is true, then you are all set to carry on with the low carb five day, two day phase shift regimen. By carefully monitoring how your body reacts to the carb level you are on and then making any necessary adjustments in carb intake, you will eventually arrive at that magic dietary carb level that is just right for you. It's important to realize that the Metabolic Diet is not a static process but a dynamic progression in which you have to be actively involved in order for it to work. If you take an interactive part in the process you will discover enough about yourself and your metabolism to achieve your fondest body weight and fat loss goals.

The initial part of the Metabolic Diet in which we determine just how your body functions under carb deprivation, is meant to be a testing ground for a person's capability for utilizing fat as a primary fuel. Those who are efficient fat oxidizers will do very well in this phase of the diet. Those who aren't may find that they will not be able to cope as well on this strict part of the diet and will do much better as the carb levels are raised in subsequent weeks.

The Metabolic Diet is designed to be a phase shift diet. That is, the weekdays are lower carb, while the weekend is higher carb. However, that is not the way it works in the first two weeks.

The best way by far to approach the first two weeks is to stay low carb for the first 12 days and then carb up on Saturday and/or Sunday. Doing it this way will give your body the incentive to make the shift from burning carbs to burning fat as its primary fuel. It will also tell you very quickly if you are totally unsuited for bottom level low carbing.

The Metabolic Diet – The Basic Steps

1. Replace the carbs you are eating now with protein and fat – do not change the calorie level at first.
2. At first, stick to the low carb phase for a full 12 days before beginning the high carb phase.
3. End carb loading the minute you start smoothing out.
4. Once you are fat adapted, change the calorie level depending on the training phase you are in.

Strict Or Assessment Phase

The Number of Grams of Carbs Allowed and the Percentage of Calories to Come From Fat, Protein and Carbs.

	Carbohydrate Intake	% Fat	% Protein	% Carbs
Weekday Maximum	30 Grams	40 – 60%	40 – 50%	4 – 10%
Weekend (12-48 Hour Carb Load)	No Real Limit	20 – 40%	15 – 30%	35 – 60%

The initial, adaptation phase of the Metabolic Diet is really quite simple. It calls for a dedicated higher fat/high protein/low-carb diet from Monday all the way through to the following Friday (a total of 12 days) before carbing up.

THE FIRST TWO WEEKS

- The Metabolic Shift Occurs From Lower Carb and Higher Fat Intake.
- 5 days is enough – as shown in recent research.
- 12 days is better.
- First carb load best on the second weekend.

During that time, except for those who are exceptionally uncomfortable (fatigue, weakness etc.), you will be limited to 30 grams of carbohydrates maximum per day. Fat should be set at roughly 50-60 percent and protein set at 30-40 percent. Follow this criteria during the initial 12-day phase of the diet and for the ensuing 5 weekdays of following weeks, assuming you are biochemically suited to this low level of carbs.

GUIDELINES FOR THE STRICT OR ASSESSMENT PHASE

- 50—60 % fat
- 30—40 % protein
- 30 grams carbohydrates

Then, come the second Saturday and subsequent Saturdays, you perform the big turnaround. You go through a higher carb phase of the diet and do the big carb up anywhere from 12 to 48 hours over the weekend and following weekends. Set your fat intake at 25-40 percent, your protein intake at 5-30 percent and carb intake at 35-55 percent. As we will see further, these levels should be adjusted to match and maximize individual body chemistry and needs.

The whole process is very similar to what athletes call "carbohydrate loading". You hit the carbs relatively heavily and this allows you to be very sociable in the dietary sense. You can eat those foods you have been missing during the week.

Guidelines For The Carb-Loading Period

- 25-40 % fat
- 15-30 % protein
- 35-55 % carbs

Basically what we are doing here in the initial or adaptation phase is limiting carbs during the first two weeks. Then, all of a sudden, the second weekend hits and you are stuffing yourself with carbohydrates. Insulin levels will rise dramatically. In fact, it's been shown that the higher fat/low-carb diet phase of the diet makes the insulin response to the high carbs even greater than it normally would be.[41,42]

The first thing your body does in response to this exaggerated carb loading is stuff the muscles with glycogen and begin to firm up. This is the portion of the diet that insures you will have an attractive foundation and not just a softened shell to shape when all that fat comes off. You will find yourself rather relaxed during this period because all those carbs will be raising serotonin in your body.

But once you get back into your regular routine Monday you will quickly find yourself energized and ready to take on the world. If you are exercising (and you should be) you will find yourself feeling especially upbeat, healthy and motivated.

During both Monday and Tuesday your system will be working hard, burning off all the increased glycogen and you gained over the weekend, and continuing to burn fatty acids. Overall you will experience a rise in fat burning and body shaping potential. Then, Wednesday to Friday, with glycogen limited again you will depend much more on your primary fat burning metabolism to maximize fat loss and body toning.

Needless to say, your body goes through a big transition weekly with this diet, whether or not you stick to the strict carb levels or increase your dietary carbs to a level where you function best. That is why it's important to know when to stop on the weekend. If you find that you have an unlimited appetite on the weekend, that is OK. You will kick the insulin into gear that much faster. But you must be careful. Some people will have a tendency to begin laying down bodyfat faster than others.

That is why you have to be aware of the point at which you begin to feel puffy and bloated. This point will vary greatly from person to person. Some people will feel hardly any response in appetite from the increased insulin. Others, however, will experience wide insulin swings and find themselves hungry and eating all the time.

That is why I list 12-48 hours as the carb load on the weekends. This could be cut back to even less than 12 hours for people whose appetites become insatiable or for people who tend to begin laying down bodyfat relatively early in the carb loading phase. The important thing is knowing when you have had enough. When you start feeling puffy and bloated and can even sense the fat coming on, it's time to go back to your weekday high fat/low carb routine.

SHORT AND LONG-TERM LOADING ON WEEKENDS

Depending on your response might want to load on low glycemic carbs for 48 hours, or perhaps only 12 hours using high glycemic carbs. Or anything in between.

Granted, it may take you awhile to learn to know your body and realize when it's telling you it's time to change phases. This point will vary widely from person to person and, while it may be easy for one person to interpret body cues, it may be harder for another. If you are having trouble with this, make the change earlier in the weekend and see how you look and feel the next week. As always, patience is the order of the day. Experience will eventually teach you to interpret your body very well and know when you are putting on fat.

Also, keep in mind that the percentages listed in the boxes for fat, protein and carb consumption are optimal numbers. If you have never done any real diet planning before, you may have a bit of trouble reaching them at first. If so, do not worry. By shooting for the 30-gram carbohydrate limitation and 40% minimum fat level in the diet during the early weeks, you will make the "metabolic shift" necessary for initial success.

The First Month

In fact, we do not want you making a lot of changes in your diet in the early weeks. Any diet, even the strict or assessment part of the Metabolic Diet, is going to be hard enough to adapt to. So do not change the amount of calories you are eating. Do not get into some serious bodyshaping regimen or otherwise make it hard on yourself. In these first weeks, simply concentrate on picking a certain calorie level you'd like to work at and then getting used to replacing the carbohydrates you eat with fat and protein.

Don't Count Calories at First

It's most important to go through the Metabolic Shift from a primarily carbohydrate burning metabolism to a fat burning one. This involves an activation of the enzymes and mechanisms involved in lipolysis, beta-oxidation of fats, ketone utilization by the CNS and other tissues, and gluconeogenesis.

Starving Yourself Is Counter Productive

The effects of cutting calories too much exaggerates fatigue and other symptoms that may be blamed on the Metabolic Shift.

If you are having trouble determining if you are at the initial 40% minimum fat level (the level of fat in the usual North American diet), focus your diet on meat dishes. This should insure that you are getting enough fat. Above all, the most important thing in the early days of the diet is to determine if you can make the "metabolic shift" to become a fat-burning machine. Do not do anything fancy until you have gone through the shift.

To insure that you go through the "metabolic shift" as quickly and efficiently as possible, do not carb load during the first weekend. If you can, continue the higher fat/low carb phase during that time.

Let me repeat this because it's important. I want you to begin the higher fat/low carb phase of the diet on a Monday. Then continue that phase, if you can, all the way through the first weekend and second week. On the second Saturday following the beginning of the diet, you will do your first carb loading. By beginning the diet with 12 days of high fat/low carb consumption, the metabolic shift will occur quickly, and with certainty, in those who are or can become efficient fat oxidizers.

Hypothetically, some dieters may decide to begin the diet on Wednesday and then immediately begin carb loading two days later. This isn't close to enough time to make the metabolic shift. Do not do it.

If you go the first 12 days on the higher fat/low carb cycle before performing a carbohydrate load you will be fine. It may be a little difficult, but it will get the job done. Doing it this way will ensure that the Assessment Phase accurately assesses whether or not you can function efficiently on dramatically reduced carbs.

However, if you find that going the 12 days is a bit too rough, then shorten it to as little as five days. A recent study has shown that 5 days is enough for most people to fat adapt.[43] The authors of the study concluded that "5 days of exposure to a high-fat, low-CHO diet caused clear changes in fuel substrate utilization during submaximal exercise and that this fat adaptation persisted through a full day carbohydrate load. At least some of these changes were independent of CHO availability because enhanced capacity for fat oxidation persisted despite restoration of muscle glycogen stores." A follow-up study by the same center confirmed the effects of a high-fat diet and CHO restoration on metabolism.[44] So going 5 days isn't all that bad as long as you stay steady on the 5 day, 2 day shift for at least a month.

Fat Adaptation

The Crux Of The Metabolic Diet

- Study below shows that fat adaptation occurs after five days of being on the Metabolic Diet and persists during one day of carbing up.

  Burke L. et al. Effect of fat adaptation and carbohydrate restoration on metabolism and performance during prolonged cycling. J Appl Physiol 89; 2413-2421.

How And When To Increase Dietary Carbohydrates

I have found it usually takes about three to four weeks on the phase shift part of the Metabolic Diet to see if we can survive and thrive on this low level of dietary carbs or if we need more carbs throughout or just at one time or another. However, for the sake of assessing whether or not the strict Metabolic Diet suits you I decided to do it 2 weeks at a time. If, after the first two weeks you feel OK, then you merely carry on with the 5+ days at 30 grams and 1-2 days in the higher carb phase.

If you are mildly to moderately tired and otherwise affected then you go through another 2 week assessment phase to see if things even out. If you are severely affected then you go on to one of the variation diets where you selectively take in more carbs depending on when you are feeling punk.

If you feel good from Saturday to Wednesday and start to get tired and generally unwell by the time Thursday rolls around, then a Wednesday carb-spike day should do the trick. So on Wednesday you should increase your carbs to at least 100 grams and usually more. You might try incorporating between 0.5 to 1 gram per pound of bodyweight of carbohydrates and see how you respond.

If you are OK most of the time but just do not have enough energy for your workouts, then you might try taking in around 50 to 100 grams of carbs after your training. You can vary the amount of carbs you use after exercise by using anywhere from 10 to 150 grams and see what works for you. The type of carbohydrate you use also makes a difference in this case. For various reasons I have found that the use of a combination of high glycemic and low glycemic carbs works best.

One word of caution, do not take any carbs prior to working out. That is because carbs at that time will decrease GH and IGF-1 production and effect, increase insulin and decrease the use of bodyfat as an primary energy source during training. The ideal pre-workout supplement is my Resolve (see below), which has no carbs but is meant, among several other things, to selectively increase growth hormone and insulin simultaneously to maximize their synergistic anabolic effects while minimizing insulin adverse effects on lipolysis and free fatty acid oxidation.

If you are tired and feel bad for most of the low carb weekdays then we can try and double the carb intake to 60 grams per day on the weekdays to see if this helps. If that doesn't help we then increase the carb intake by 30 grams per day once a week for as many weeks as it takes for you to feel normal and function optimally.

Most people who have to increase their daily carbs usually level off between 100 and 200 grams per day. I have found that about one-half to one gram of dietary carbs per pound bodyweight per day is the norm in those who are relatively poor fat oxidizers. In a small number of cases it may be necessary to work up to as much as 3 grams of carbs per pound of body weight, depending on the individual and the activity that he or she is involved in.

When you have to increase the level of carbs in your diet it will take a while before you discover what your carb set point is (see Problem-Solving Guide). I have found that it takes people about two months on the average to find their ideal dietary carb level. Once you discover your Metabolic Set Point, you can fix your diet at that level for several months while you work on changing your body composition.

Varying Your Daily Calories

Some people find it difficult to stick to a daily calorie limit but may find it easier to work on a weekly calorie limit so that on some days they can take in more calories while on others less. If you are strict about your weekly calorie intake there is no reason not to count calories on a weekly rather than a daily level. In fact some bodybuilders find that they make even better progress by keeping the body guessing rather than having it adapt to fixed daily calorie intake.

Varying Calories

- Work on weekly calorie intake and vary carbs every other day or every third day or whatever suits you.
- For example, total weekday calories is set at 3,000*5 = 15,000 calories. Can take 2,000 one day, 3,000 next, 5,000 next, 2,000 next and then on the last weekday take in remaining 3,000.

Problem-Solving Guide

Steps to take in determining your carbohydrate set point – the ideal level of dietary carbs for your body.

By following this short guide you can determine just how much and when to take the carbs your body needs to function optimally.

If you are feeling fine:

1. I am starting on a 2-Week Assessment Phase of the Strict Metabolic Diet to see how well I do on the 30g Carb Weekday, 150g+ Carb Weekends.
2. I have been following the 30g Carb Weekday, 150g+ Carb Weekends for 2 weeks now and I am doing well. What do I do now?
3. You are an efficient fat burner and your system has made the shift successfully. At this point you can start with the weekly 5 day 2 day phase shifts, limiting your carbs during the week and then increasing your carbs over 1 to 2 days of the weekend.

If you are feeling tired:

1. I am feeling tired and I need some help with the carbohydrate part of my diet.
2. I only have low to moderate tiredness at this time so I will do another 2-week Assessment Phase to see how well I do?
3. Yes carry on with another assessment phase. In most cases this extra 12 days usually results in a success on the diet and a disappearance of the tiredness.
4. I am still tired after the second 2 week assessment phase. What do I do now?
5. The next step is to determine when you are tired and increase your carb intake appropriately.
6. I am tired all the time.
7. Increase your daily carb intake by 30 grams per day until the tiredness disappears. Once you have reached a level of carbs that works for you try to slowly cut back on the daily carbs until the tiredness returns. Then jack the carbs up slightly until you feel normal.
8. I have a mid-Late Week' tiredness, so what do I need to do?
9. Try a mid-Week Carb Spike' of an additional 120g+ of carbs just on Wednesday and see how well you do.

10. I did the mid-Week Carb Spike' and/or increased my daily carbs so I am not tired normally but now I lack energy during training?.

11. You need to take from 30 up to 100g of carbs half an hour after training to combat this lack of energy on training days. This should increase your muscle glycogen levels for subsequent training days and give you all the energy you need to train.

12. I tried increasing my carb intake during training but I am still lacking energy during training, so what can I do?

13. Increase your daily carbohydrate intake by 30 grams a day until the tiredness disappears.

TROUBLE SHOOTING GUIDE & EXPERIMENTING WITH FOODS

Increasing carbs:

➲ Increase daily carb intake by 30 grams or more at a time.

➲ Midweek Carb Spike – a few hours to all day

➲ Carbs added after training. Spike in muscle glycogen, intramuscular fatty acids and protein synthesis.

What To Eat

I will provide some information on what to eat in this book but for more specifics, and especially for over 175 pages of information on foods, including various tables, comprehensive calorie, protein, carb and fat charts, and extensive example diets at every calorie level you will need to get a copy of the more than 500 page Metabolic Diet. Some of this information is also available on my site **www.MetabolicDiet.com**. For example, the two-week sample diets can be found at this address: **http://www.metabolicdiet.com/mdiet_index.htm**.

WHAT TO EAT

➲ Weekdays – Any high protein, low carb foods – meats, fish, eggs, cheeses, low carb vegetables – most except big beans, corn, carrots, peas.

➲ Fiber in all forms – both soluble and insoluble. Cover this in Nutritional Supplement Presentation.

➲ Weekends, almost anything goes. Time limited. Go back to the low carb phase as soon as you start smoothing out.

During the weekdays, there are plenty of options for high fat/high protein/low carb foods available. Virtually any meat is OK, and most of you will focus on steak, hamburger, pork and other red meats on the diet. In addition, venison, fish (of great importance as we will see later), lamb, shrimp, lobster, chicken, turkey, and other white meats are also OK. So are canned sardines, tuna, shrimp, herring and anchovies.

Almost any kind of cheese is fair game as well. Use the full fat and non-skimmed milk varieties. Keep in mind that cheese spreads, cottage and ricotta cheese are higher in carbohydrates. Brie, Camembert, Muenster, Gruyere and Monterey jack are very low in carbs and good for the diet.

Whole eggs are great. Deviled eggs can be a good snack food to keep in the refrigerator to use. Butter and poly- and monounsaturated oils are fine (subject to certain restrictions outlined below). Nuts and seeds like walnuts and sunflower seeds are also good, but keep track of the carbs. So are condiments such as salt, vinegar, oil, and mayonnaise, although we urge you to use oil (especially olive oil) and vinegar dressing most of the time. Most other commercial salad dressings are in the vicinity of 7 percent carbohydrates.

Sugar is going to be a problem for people with a sweet tooth. You can end up craving it, especially during the assessment phase of the diet. Look to appease any cravings along this line with low carb drinks and desserts with artificial sweeteners. However, avoid sorbitol and fructose – remember sugar free doesn't necessarily mean carb free. Make sure and check the labels. Diet soft drinks are fine.

You can also put sugar free Jell-O (no carbs, uses artificial sweetener) to good use. Topping it with carb-free whipped cream may be just what you are looking for to gain control. It has no carbs and many people on the Metabolic Diet have found it quite successful in appeasing any cravings. Just be sure to check the labels on whipping cream containers to make sure carbs haven't been added.
Another factor to consider is that, even if you have cravings, you are only putting off satisfying them until the weekend. You can eat basically anything then. We are just partitioning or separating foods here. We are not saying you cannot have lasagna. You just have to wait for the weekend. That is a lot better than other diets where you are basically stranded on Low-Fat or, in some cases, Low-Carb Island for the rest of your life.

This can also work for you psychologically. Foods you love can give you a goal. Just get to the weekend and you can have that slice of apple pie. You are giving yourself something to look forward to and it can even be fun. This doesn't present the kind of depression and boredom you get eating the same thing over and over, week after week, month after month. You do not have to come up with an elaborate set of recipes to keep yourself sane.

When you get to the weekend, do what you want! Fill up the tank on the foods you want. Satisfy those cravings. Some people will go overboard at the beginning of the diet and eat until they are nearly sick. Most will overdo it to some degree, but this is fine. It gets easier as you go.

Once they have been on the diet awhile, most people will not have that strong desire for ice cream or onion rings anymore. They will eat them but they will not pig out and, as they start adjusting their diets and dialing them in for maximum progress, they will begin to see some real improvement and acquire some real knowledge about the way their body works and how adjustments can be made to achieve their goals.

The Metabolic Diet can also be adjusted depending on special circumstances. For example the changes you can make if your serum cholesterol is not where it should be – see section above on Your Cholesterol.

Here's Just A Few Of The High Fat/Low Carb Weekday Foods You Can Eat On the Metabolic Diet

➲ Steak	➲ Hamburger	➲ Sausage	➲ Venison
➲ Salmon	➲ Lamb	➲ Shrimp	➲ Lobster
➲ Chicken	➲ Turkey	➲ Tuna	➲ Herring
➲ Anchovies	➲ Cheese*	➲ Eggs	➲ Butter
➲ Oils**	➲ Walnuts	➲ Pot Roast	➲ Pastrami
➲ Bacon	➲ Mayonnaise	➲ Salt	➲ Diet Soda
➲ Jell-O***	➲ Hamburger	➲ Sunflower Seeds	

* Full Fat/Low-Carb
** Poly and monounsaturated fats such as is found in nuts, olive oil, flax seed oil
*** Sugar-free

KEYS TO EARLY DIET SUCCESS

1. Do not worry about calories
2. Take a fiber supplement
3. Watch for hidden carbs
4. Do not mix diets
5. The first week is the toughest – Stick It Out

When To Eat Your Carbs

A real question that comes into play on the higher fat/low carb portion of the Metabolic Diet is when to eat your carbs during the day. Some people spread them out. Others get most of them in one meal. Again, the answer has to do with personal preference. You can eat your carbs at any time of day and it will not matter, as long as you do not go above the 30-gram carb limit.

Some people find eating their carbs throughout the day makes them hungrier and lazier. They will feel sluggish. They get that "turkey dinner syndrome" where they finish and all they feel like doing is laying on the couch. This isn't good, especially for a busy person who needs to feel motivated and energized during the day.

When To Eat Your Carbs

Can be flexible:

- Throughout the day in form of low glycemic vegetables.
- At one time as a reward.
- After training.

Many people believe that our eating patterns have become counterproductive in modern society. The average American eats a lot of carbs during the day and the insulin and serotonin responses we talked about earlier can become very pronounced. At times of the day when we need to be productive and alert, in the early afternoon for instance, we will be sleepy and lethargic from all those carbs and the resulting hormone and neurotransmitter rush.

For those people it would be better to save the carbs for later in the day. That is what a lot of people do on the Metabolic Diet. They will keep the carbs minimum during the day and find their energy levels much increased as a result. Then they will come home at night and have the bulk of their carbs with dinner. The carbs at dinner will find them unwinding in the evening hours, relaxing and sleeping like a baby at night.

It's interesting to note that one of the trends in business today is toward a more streamlined lunch. Those huge, three-martini lunches are no longer the norm. Executives and employees are eating and drinking more sensibly in the middle of the day and finding productivity rising as a result. This comes not only from time saved at lunch but also from the improved attitude that comes with getting rid of all those carbs and alcohol at noon.

Another good time to take your carbs is after exercising. For a few hours after exercise there is a window of opportunity when hormonal factors are just right for rebuilding muscle.

Taking carbohydrates during this time period spikes insulin levels and increases protein synthesis, thus maximizing the effects exercise has on strengthening and toning your body.

A few carboholics who are on my diet reserve their carbs for the evening. They eat almost no carbs during the day so they can have their 30 or so grams at night in the form of ice cream or a chocolate bar. That is OK as long as you do not go over your daily carb quota.

Experiment

Personal experience and individual body chemistry will have a great deal to do with how you structure the diet. Different people will have differing responses to the carb-loading portion of the diet. The length of that carb-loading period may vary greatly as a result.

The 30-gram carbohydrate limit is also not written in stone. It serves as a good guide and should be adhered to when beginning the diet, but some people may find that they can later increase carb intake to as high as 50 grams per day and still do fine. Others may find that anything over 20 will make them feel sluggish. I have also found that people on the higher calorie diets, mainly seen in the Mass phase, can take in a tad over 30 grams and still be OK and we have accounted for this in the higher calorie sample diets. Once you have made the "metabolic shift" and made the diet a part of your life, you can experiment to find what works best for you.

EXPERIMENT

- The Metabolic Diet is all about adjusting the diet to suit your metabolism.
- As such, experimenting to see what works best for you is the cornerstone of the Metabolic Diet.
- Can do it on a weekly basis so that each week can be a learning experience
- Vary protein, fat and carbs and the times you take them.

Fat levels may also be experimented with to some degree. Some may find optimum results going as low as 30 percent fat on the diet, but you must beware. You cannot go too low, especially at first when your body is going through the shift from utilizing fats instead of carbs as its primary fuel.

Taking in a lot of protein helps, but not without the fat. Without enough dietary fat, even if you are limiting your carb intake, your body will not “learn” how to use fat as a primary fuel. Your body basically says, "I am not going to get rid of this stuff because I may need it down the road." Limit fat in your diet and your body wants to lay it on as a way of keeping it around. You end up cutting dietary fat but adding bodyfat.[45] A bodybuilder recently told me that he tried to make the shift to burning bodyfat as the main fuel (one of the goals behind the Metabolic Diet) by going on a high protein low-carb, low-fat diet, basically an all protein diet. He began doing the egg whites, boiled chicken breasts and canned tuna in water thing, but with no carbs, and, while he ended up losing fat, his body shriveled up. He looked awful.

The fact is that your body needs the fat to adjust to burning fat while at the same time sparing muscle. Increasing dietary fat intake will increase your body's use of both dietary and bodyfat as a primary fuel by increasing the levels of enzymes needed for increased fat breakdown and decreasing the enzymes involved in storing bodyfat. The bottom line is that you are basically losing bodyfat by increasing the fat in your diet.

So do not worry too much about your overall fat percentages because they usually will take care of themselves unless you mistakenly, at least at first, try to limit your fat intake. Of course you can make some adjustments depending on how you are responding to the diet, but be careful. Remember, if you do not give the body enough fat you will not make the shift to a fat-based metabolism and your body will lose its shape, which is exactly what you do not want.

This may sound like nonsense, but it's not. Give the bodyfat and it will use that fat and burn off bodyfat. When you are fat adapted the body is into metabolizing fat as a primary fuel so that even if you cut back on dietary fat, your body will still burn fat and spare muscle, only this time it will get the fat it needs from your bodyfat.

One of the good things about this diet is that you do not have to become paranoid and keep elaborate charts to get that proper amount of fat in your diet. In fact, if you are diligent about eating your red meat and other animal food — bacon, ham, steak, burger, fish, etc., and in using olive oil — you shouldn't have to worry about hitting the 40-60% fat and 40—50% protein ratios listed above. It will naturally happen.

Again, it's important to realize that individual experimentation will play a large role in aspects of the Metabolic Diet. The diet should be varied to provide the optimum level of performance and success for the individual. We are all different to some degree according to body chemistry and needs. No two human beings are alike. No two human beings will implement this diet entirely alike, either. As you make the diet a part of your daily lifestyle, experiment with it to find the best way to execute the diet for you.

Eating Out

I have a friend who's been on the Metabolic Diet for several years now. Frequently we go out to eat together during the week and he's got the right approach down to a fine art. He looks the waiter in the eye and says "I want a T-bone steak and nothing else!" Most often the waiter will look at him and say, "But you get a baked potato, vegetables, bread . . ."

"AND NOTHING ELSE," he breaks in and repeats. Waiters may have a little difficulty understanding this at first but usually, with repetition, the point will sink in.

The fact is that my friend wisely doesn't want the extras on his plate. He doesn't need the temptation. The meat is fine by him. He feels great, sticks to his diet and feels good when he's through. If he eats that potato, bread and coleslaw he will not. Order what you want regardless of what the waiter says. If he tries to tell you that you are wasting your money, tell him he's wasting his time.

During the week, you should be staying away from those carbohydrate foods so keep them out of sight and out of mind. Leave them off your plate; otherwise, you might be tempted to "sample" them.

On the weekend, everything is different. All that bread, potato and salad are fair game. Depending on how you have got your diet structured, you can order them twice. Just keep them off your plate during the week.

EATING OUT

- Only a problem during weekdays
- Be specific when ordering so that the waiter doesn't bring carbs to the table to tempt you.
- If it's a problem, don't eat out until you have more control.

Doing It Your Way

Varying Carb Intake

Besides experimenting with different foods and schedules there are various other ways you can fine-tune the diet so that it fits in with your metabolic abilities. While all of us posses the ability to use fat as our primary fuel, some are more able than others are. This is because we all have different genetic capabilities and while some have it in them to be efficient fat burners, some of us do not.

You will know after the first few weeks if you are among the few who have difficulty adjusting and using fats as a primary fuel. These people tend to have a tougher time making the switch, can feel tired and are easily exhausted by physical activity. It seems that they just run out of gas shortly after their weekend carbup.
That is because they are metabolism prefers carbs to fats and cannot seem to make do on the five day, two day shift. During the weekend they carb load and feel OK for the first few

days of the week but when their glycogen reserves are used up they often feel like they have been hit by a truck.

Just because your body prefers carbs and cannot operate as well on fats doesn't mean you have to abandon the Metabolic Diet. It just means you have to change the amount and timing of your carb intake so that the maximum amount of fat is burned along with the necessary carbs. If you can find the minimum carb intake that you need to function normally then you can benefit from the Metabolic Diet.

Now lets say you have done the first two months but still do not feel right, even though you are using the right supplements and doing everything right. You are may be tired much of the time, especially Wednesday to Friday and your training may be suffering because you have lost the enthusiasm and stamina you once had. It's time to fine-tune your carb intake. You can do this in one of several ways.

Increasing Your Weekday Carb Intake

One way is to gradually increase your daily carb intake (by about 10 grams per day) until you reach a level where your symptoms improve. For most people that level will be somewhere between 50 to 100 grams of carbs per day.

It's just as important to time your carb intake, as it is to increase the amount of carbs you take in. Besides finding the baseline carb level you also have to find the best time to take these carbs. For people who have to raise their carb levels I find the best time to take the extra carbs is before and after training. For example you might want to take 20 to 30 grams of carbs prior to training, along with the pretraining supplement, and another 20 to 30 grams after training along with your post training meal or meal replacement powder.

On the other hand, you might find that your low point is in the evening after you have worked a long day. In this case a carb spike right after work might be your best bet. Or you just might want to spread out the extra carbs throughout the day. Whatever works best for you keeping in mind that you are looking for the least amount of daily carbs to do the job.

Another important factor here is the kinds of carbs. High glycemic carbs are absorbed very quickly and give rise to a rapid insulin rise. In most cases increasing the lower glycemic carbs by increasing your vegetable intake is the best route to take. For most people doubling or even tripling the carb intake in this way helps them over the low carb hump, and doesn't seem to affect their weight and fat loss while at the same time they do not experience carb cravings. If these same people take in carbs from other sources, say from dairy products or high glycemic foods, it can stop their weight and fat loss and make them hungry.

For some people, eating higher glycemic carbs may work best prior to and after training. Everybody is different so it's important to experiment with different foods. But be careful.

Keep an eye on how you look and the progress you are making. If you are losing ground then it's not for you and you have to rethink what you are doing.

The Midweek Carb Spike

Some people may find that what they need is a midweek "carb spike". This replenishes their glycogen stores and holds them over until the weekend. You can do the carb spike in several ways.

One way is to dramatically increase your carb intake for that day by either taking it in all at once (like a pancake and syrup feed) or spread it out over the day, using either high and/or low glycemic foods. One popular way is to take in a mini-carb load lasting an hour on Wednesday morning. During the "carb spike" most people concentrate on loading up with high glycemic foods and take in between 200 to 800, sometimes as many as 1000 calories in that hour. Once you have had your mid week carb feed, you should head right back to low carb land.

For some people, a midweek jolt of carbs can be very productive for those interested in advanced body shaping or building. The increased blood sugar and subsequent insulin spike will increase muscle and liver glycogen dramatically, give you an extra energy "kick" and drive amino acids into muscle cell for increased development. As long as you go right back to the Metabolic Diet, you will avoid lying on unwanted fat.

In all cases where you increase your carb intake during the week it's important that you subsequently curb some of your carb intake over the weekend. That way you will not be overdoing your long-term carb intake. For example you might only want to carb load one day over the weekend or even skip the weekend carb up altogether.

Short-term Loading On Weekends

On the weekends you are usually pretty free to take in whatever foods you like. In general you will be increasing both your calories and carbs without too much worry over what kinds of foods you eat. On the other hand there are some caveats.

For some two days of carb loading may be too much, especially if you go overboard and eat everything in sight. One of my male patients used to keep his calorie level at about 2000 calories per day during to weekdays and jump to 10,000 calories per day the weekend. Needless to say we had to curtail his carb overload on the weekends so he could reach his weight and fat loss goals.

Also some people can get pretty sensitive to carbs and find that after carb loading for one day they just do not feel right. They bloat out, feel tired, and just do not function very well. In these cases it's best to just carb up for one day or even part of one day and then get back on the higher fat/low-carb diet. This will make the diet a 6-day low carb, 1-day high carb experience, but if this works for you then it's the way to go. Again, the length of carb loading depends on the individual. The important thing is to experiment with the length of your weekend carb load and learn what works best for you.

Eating foods very high in glycemic value with less fat will generally lead to a shorter, more intense carb load. You will almost certainly start to lose tone and retain water sooner, often before the 24-hour mark. By using lower glycemic carbs, or combining foods (such as pasta mixed in with protein and fat), you will take longer to load. You may want to experiment with both of these approaches to see what works best.

Keep in mind that it's important to document aspects of the diet and their effects on your body. It may be inconvenient or even painful, but if you are interested in getting the most out of your efforts, you have got to chart your progress and the ways you respond to changes in the diet. Make notes to yourself on when you begin to smooth out during the weekend, what you were eating, how many calories you were eating and any other essential information.

Keeping your own diet log will give you a record of what you have done and give you added confidence with the moves you make in training and diet. This is the way you will really dial in the time when you look best and how to get that look. You may back off on the documentation after being on the diet for some time and becoming familiar with it, but you will still want to make at least weekly notes on your findings as you proceed.

Long-term Loading On Weekends

Some people will cheat in the other direction on this diet and they will pay for it. They get to Thursday and then suddenly decide they are going to start their carb load on Friday. They continue it on through Sunday and, guess what? Their body shifts back to a carbohydrate metabolism. Three days is too much. At that point, you are running a real risk of losing the fat burning advantage this diet gives you. Long-term carb loading is not a good idea.
But the higher fat/low-carb diet is forgiving. If you are at a birthday party in the middle of the week and do not want to be anti-social, you can have that piece of cake. Likewise, business or social conditions may warrant a high carb meal during the week on occasion. Do not worry about it. As long as you get right back on the higher fat/low-carb diet you will not find your body shifting back. After you have been on the diet for a while it will usually take at least three days of continuous carbs for the metabolism to shift back.

In fact, the longer you are on the Metabolic Diet, the more time it seems to take to go back to a carbohydrate metabolism. For those who have been on the diet for years, it may eventually become as difficult to make the switch back to burning glucose for energy, as it was to go through the metabolic shift to become a fat-burner.

The Metabolic Diet suppresses the glycolytic pathway used by the body when carbs are the primary energy source. At the same time, the lipolytic (fat burning) pathway is activated. The longer you are on the diet, the more carbohydrate loading it seems to require to activate the glycolytic pathway fully again. Even if you go out on the road and you are forced to change diets for a week, you can generally return to the diet without going through another metabolic shift if you have become a the Metabolic Diet veteran.

The Metabolic Diet may even be accident-proof. One Metabolic dieter who'd been on the diet several months began limiting most of his carbohydrate consumption to a bowl of ice cream at the end of the day. Several months later he suddenly took a close look at the package and found he was eating double the carbs he thought he was. Yet he never spilled back over to the glucose metabolism. It seems that, through the suppression of the glycolytic enzyme, his body had set a new level of tolerance for carbohydrates.

Not that we suggest you double your carb intake during the weekdays. This is just to say that the Metabolic Diet doesn't make you pay dearly for any mistake. After shifting over on the diet, it will generally take a minimum of 3 days of carbs to do serious metabolic damage.

Varying Calories

Many bodybuilders have found that if they do the same workout every day, their body becomes used to it and no longer respond. They do not get stronger. They will plateau. You may eventually find this to be true in your own exercise program.

It's the same with the Metabolic Diet. If you eat the same exact amount of calories every day, you may eventually start to lose the effect of the diet. That is why you should try to do some varying of calories on a day-to-day basis. Stairstep them. If 2000 calories a day is your goal, try taking 3000 calories one day, 1000 the next, 2500 the day after that and so forth. Count your calories on a weekly basis instead of daily. Be unpredictable. Do not let your body get used to the same caloric intake daily. By doing this you keep the body guessing so that it doesn't make some adverse hormonal changes, or drop the basal metabolic rate (BMR) to accommodate the drop in calories.

STAIRSTEPPING – 3,000 CALORIE DIET

- Monday 3,500 Calories
- Tuesday 2,000 Calories
- Wednesday 3,000 Calories
- Thursday 4,000 Calories
- Friday 2,500 Calories

Total 15,000 Calories (3,000/day)

You can also vary those calories on the weekend. A good rule of thumb at the beginning is to increase calories no more than 25 percent over your weekday allotment but, once experienced with the diet, you are on your own. However, you do have to be careful. If you take in a lot of calories, especially the high glycemic variety, you may find yourself laying down fat very quickly.

Extreme Variance

Some have tried extreme increases in calories during the weekend and experienced success. Those dieters who want to maximize lean body mass and lose bodyfat rather than lose weight mainly use this method. They get to Saturday and intuitively sense that it's time to shake their metabolism loose. They will take in up to 10,000 calories on Saturday, maybe cut it in half on Sunday, and experience a huge insulin spike. They will get a big effect as far as bodyshaping but, because they go right back on the higher fat/low-carb diet on Monday, insulin will be limited before it begins to encourage much laying down of fat.

The dieter may end up gaining up to 10 pounds or so from the extra sugar and water, but the high fat/low-carb diet will find him dropping the water weight quickly as the week progresses. By Friday, he will have increased weight to a strategic degree but will not have overdone it, and the increase will be maximum muscle and minimum fat.

Low Protein Weekends

After being on the diet for a while, you may want to begin treating the weekends as a high carb/higher fat exercise while paying less attention to protein. Some people who have been on the diet for an extended period have found that a weekend diet of around 40-45 percent fat, 50-55 percent carbs and only 7-10 percent protein can produce excellent results.

The added fat aids in slowing the release of glucose in the blood, thus avoiding sugar rushes or crashes that can leave you feeling spent and irritable. By using lower glycemic foods with increased dietary fat, you will also be able to extend the length of your carb load and not feel the puffiness and bloat that should signal its end. As for the protein, you are getting enough during the week to get through the weekend with no problems.

As well, studies have shown that protein utilization after relative protein restriction rebounds to higher levels than was present prior to the restriction. Studies have also shown that in times of protein depletion, the body likely conserves muscle protein and increases the burning of fat stores for energy. This adaptation is usually lost when bodyfat stores near exhaustion.[46]

In summary the weekend protein break will not have any adverse consequences on your attempts to build a more muscular body, and may in fact enhance the process of fat loss.

Follow That Instinctive Voice

If you are on a minimal calorie diet, you have got to listen to that instinctive voice in your body and do what it tells you to do. If it says eat, eat. As minimal as your caloric intake may be, you are trying to manage it not starve yourself.

This is another area where the higher fat/low-carb diet has an advantage over the competition. On the high-carb diet, if you are in a negative calorie intake situation (where your body requires more calories for weight maintenance than you are putting in), you will use up the carbs you are eating for energy very quickly. After that, the primary source for energy will be mostly protein and some fat. On the high-carb diet, you can find yourself losing a lot of muscle tone because of the body raiding protein for energy. Not so with the Metabolic Diet, where there is fat available to burn instead of protein. Protein is thus saved and so is muscle.

Remember, too, that fat is satiating. It delays the onset of hunger and you feel fuller after you eat it. You will also experience fewer cravings when you have made the metabolic shift to being a "fat burner". These characteristics can be most helpful in a situation where you are burning more calories than you are taking in.

Keys to Success on the Metabolic Diet

- Do not seek a weight loss at the beginning
- Caloric intake will vary between individuals
- Try to lose 1.5- 2 pounds weekly
- Keep track of inches as well as pounds
- Use calipers to measure bodyfat
- Weigh/measure no more than once weekly
- Do not pick an ideal weight
- Goals are 18 percent bodyfat for women/10 percent for men
- Rely on the mirror more than the scales
- Do not change your lifestyle or habits once you reach your target weight
- Experiment with caloric intake to find a proper maintenance level
- Experiment with foods

CHAPTER FIVE

Good And Bad Fats

Using Your Head

Before we get into the specifics of how best to mentally approach the Metabolic Diet, you will need to become better acquainted with its basics. Only by "using your head" to intelligently choose foods and keep yourself motivated and committed will you achieve the most progress and success.

One key to your success will be in understanding the difference between "good fats" and "bad fats", maximizing the former, minimizing the latter and eating the different kinds of fat in the proper proportions. While some of the information in this chapter may be somewhat technical, the recommendations and applications will be easy to understand and apply.

What Are Fats?

For many years, most diet gurus have been preaching the ills of dietary fat. The fact is that dietary fat is essential for good health. They are necessary for the proper absorption, transportation and function of the fat-soluble vitamins A, D, E, and K. Lipids (a general term for all types of fats) are used by the body to produce hormones and other substances than can aid good health and protect against degenerative diseases. They are also an excellent energy source, much superior to the fruits, vegetables and other carbs the Experts keep hailing at the expense of other foods.

Components of lipids known as "essential fatty acids" (EFAs) are necessary building blocks for all cell membranes in the body. They also make up many of the more intricate structures inside the cells. The retina (which turns light into nerve impulses in the eye) and nerve synapses (which join the body's individual nerve cells) rely on EFAs for structure. These are the types of fat that are essential to life.

However, there are other fats that can actually destroy good health and lead to serious problems down the road. To understand the difference between these "good fats" and "bad fats" we need to look at the basic chemical structure of fats to see how they vary.
Fats and oils (an animal or plant fat that is liquid at room temperature) are made up of a number of repeating molecular units. One molecule of fat consists of a single molecule of an alcohol called glycerol combined with three molecules of fatty acids. The fatty acids are

made up of chains of carbon and hydrogen atoms with a methyl group (3 atoms of hydrogen, one carbon) at one end, chains of carbon and hydrogen atoms in the middle, and a carboxyl group (made up of carbon, oxygen and hydrogen) at the other end. The hydrogen atoms are connected to each carbon atom and their number and position determine the degree of saturation of the fatty acid and its shape.

Figure: Saturated Fatty Acid

Figure: Unsaturated Fatty Acid

Fatty acids can be classified as either "saturated" or "unsaturated". In the diagrams above, you will note that the "saturated" fatty acids contain carbon atoms that are linked to two hydrogen atoms. They are thus "saturated" with hydrogen atoms because they are linked to as many hydrogen atoms as possible. The term "saturated fat" refers to the hydrogen atoms attached to the carbon atoms.

In the "unsaturated" diagrams above, you will note that a double bond joins several of the carbon atoms together. When a double bond is present, each carbon atom will only be attached to a single hydrogen atom. The carbon atoms are no longer connected to the maximum hydrogen atoms and are said to be "unsaturated". A "monounsaturated" fatty acid contains a single incidence of double bonds along its chain. A "polyunsaturated" fatty acid would feature two or more connections along its chain where two carbon atoms are double-bonded.

The hardness of a fat decreases with the increase in its double bonds. As a result, most of the liquid fats like vegetable and fish oils are polyunsaturated. Sometimes food producers will add hydrogen to the double bonds of a chain to make them less unsaturated in a process called "hydrogenation". In this way, vegetable oils can be hardened into shortening for use in cooking.

Stearic Acid (SA) [18:0]

```
    H H H H H H H H H H H H H H H H H
    | | | | | | | | | | | | | | | | |    //O
H - C-C-C-C-C-C-C-C-C-C-C-C-C-C-C-C-C - C
    | | | | | | | | | | | | | | | | |    \
    H H H H H H H H H H H H H H H H H     OH
```

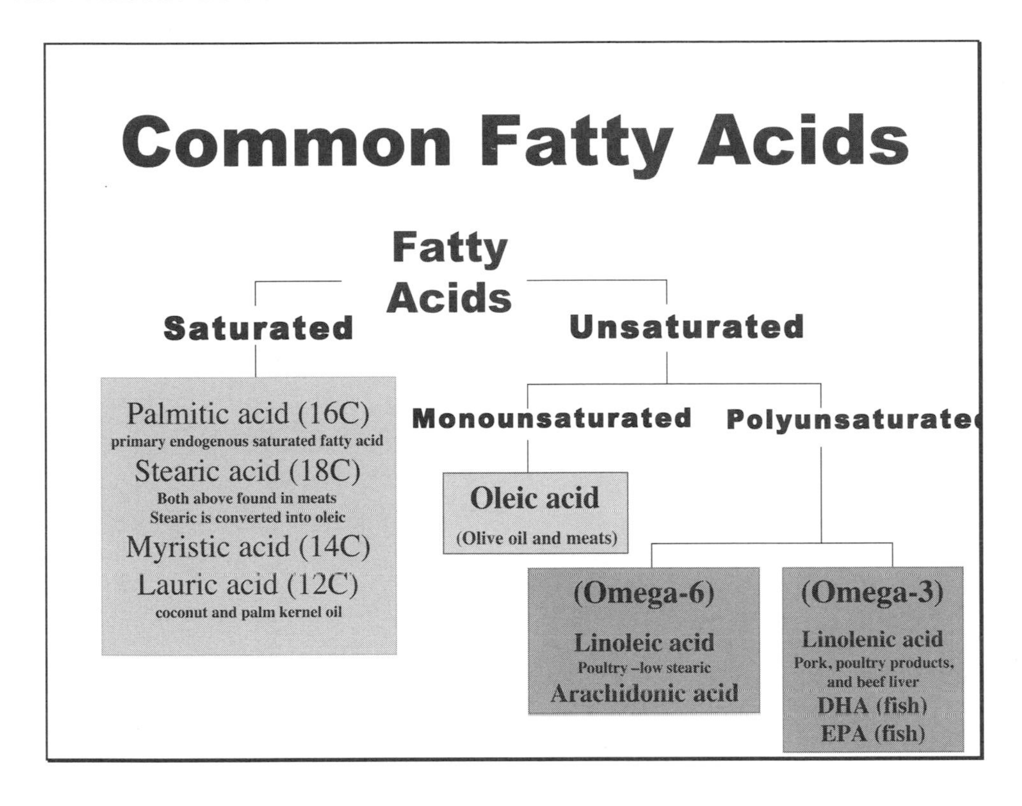

Good Fats

The two essential fatty acids linoleic acid (LA) and alpha-linolenic acid (LNA) (also called omega fats) are critical to health and must be supplied in a person's diet since the human body cannot manufacture them.

Linoleic acid is classified as an omega-6 fatty acid. Omega-6 fatty acids are polyunsaturated fatty acids that have their endmost double bond six carbon atoms away from the CH3 end of a chain. Alpha-linolenic acid is an omega-3 fatty acid. Omega-3's are polyunsaturated fatty acids with their endmost double bond three carbon atoms from the CH3 end.

Many people do not get sufficient amounts of EFAs in their diets. Getting enough LNA seems to be more of a problem. This of course can cause health problems because these EFAs are necessary for growth, the integrity of cell membranes and the synthesis of important hormone-like substances called eicosanoids.

Now this is where we have to get very technical. But bear with me; the end result of this discussion will be easy to understand recommendations that will improve your health and the effectiveness of the Metabolic Diet.

The Eicosanoids: Piecing Together The Puzzle

Eicosanoids are physiologically active metabolites of EFAs with important effects on the immune, cardiovascular and central nervous system. Amongst these are prostaglandins and arachidonic acid, from which the eicosanoids are synthesized.

Eicosanoids act locally in and around the tissues in which they are produced. Virtually all cells in the body can form some of the eicosanoids, but tissues differ in enzyme profile and consequently in the products they form. They also differ in their ability to be affected by specific eicosanoids. Eicosanoids are not stored to any degree and must be synthesized in response to immediate need.

While it would be advantageous to be able to direct eicosanoid production so that good eicosanoids would be produced deferentially to bad ones, it is difficult to do so because of the complexity of eicosanoid production, actions and metabolism. Unfortunately we do not know a lot about the dietary influences that affect the known eicosanoids and thus can make only limited use of any knowledge we do have.

For example, some of the bad eicosanoids, such as PGE2, a series two prostaglandin that increases platelet aggregation and inflammation and has adverse effects on the cardiovascular system, are derived from arachidonic acid. We could thus reason that by inhibiting the enzyme that catalyzes the synthesis of arachidonic acid, less PGE2 would be formed. As well, more metabolites would be present for forming some of the good eicosanoids such as PGE1, a series one prostaglandin that has several favorable effects on blood clotting, inflammation and the cardiovascular system.

We know that various factors such as eicosapentaenoic acid, glucagon and even cholesterol and alcohol can inhibit the formation of arachidonic acid or the formation of

Figure from "Fats that Heal Fats that Kill" by Udo Erasmus, alive books Vancouver

PGE2 from arachidonic acid. However, utilizing this knowledge to manipulate the eicosanoids is difficult since we really need more information on the complex ways these compounds are formed, act and are metabolized. Although we could possibly formulate a working game plan, it would not be written in stone and has to be validated by ongoing research.

For example, prostaglandins can be both good and bad. Unfortunately, it is difficult to stimulate the good ones and not the bad ones. If we decrease the formation of prostaglandins from arachidonic acid we inhibit the formation of both good and bad prostaglandins. Of more relevance for dieters, it is not possible to differentially stimulate the production of PGI2, which has a lipolytic action, from PGE2, which has an antilipolytic action. Both prostaglandins belong to the series 2 prostaglandins and are formed from arachidonic acid.

At present, some treatment strategies using EFAs have tentatively been formulated to try and take advantage of the good eicosanoids. For example, omega-3 fatty acids found in fish oils can decrease production of some arachidonate metabolites and increase levels of certain prostaglandins. Feeding of these fatty acids has been used as a therapeutic strategy to diminish platelet aggregation.

Confused? So are most people, especially since all the pieces to the puzzle haven't all been uncovered. The gist of trying to modify your intake of the omega 6 and omega 3 fatty acids is that we can, by the use of a special diet, direct the flow of linoleic acid to the good eicosanoids instead of the bad eicosanoids. This may be done by increasing the transformation of linoleic acid to gamma-linolenic acid (GLA) and/or supplementing GLA by using GLA-rich oils, and directing the formation of the good eicosanoids instead of arachidonic acid.

There are many factors that can inhibit the enzyme delta-6-desaturase, the enzyme responsible for the conversion of LA to GLA. These factors include LNA (the other essential fatty acid), trans fatty acids (see below), stress and viral infections. By limiting these factors, more GLA can be naturally formed from dietary LA.

As well, there are many factors that can inhibit the delta-5-desaturase enzyme, the one responsible for the formation of arachidonic acid (AA) from dihomo-gamma-linolenic acid (DGLA). These factors include glucagon and EPA. Insulin increases the formation of arachidonic acid from DGLA and thus increases the formation of the bad eicosanoids.

So, in theory, dietary practices can limit the production or transformation of arachidonic acid and encourage the production and transformation of GLA, thus maximizing the production of good eicosanoids over the bad ones. It's difficult, because we do not have many pieces of the puzzle to say if this is true. If further substantiated by research, this way of altering eicosanoid synthesis though changes in our intake of EFAs may well be one of the few coordinated practical uses of the complex scientific information on the eicosanoids. While we may not know for sure if what were doing accomplishes the changes we'd like to see, we can make certain dietary recommendations that fit in to the available research.
In the Metabolic Diet, I discourage excess carbohydrate consumption and encourage the use of good fats in the diet, including the use of fish and fish oils and sources of GLA such as evening primrose and borage seed oils. At present, this is the best we can do is to make sure that enough and the right proportion of the EFAs and other members of the omega-6 and omega-3 fatty acids are present in the diet.

The omega-3's like LNA and eicosapentaenoic and docosahexaenoic acids (known as EPA and DHA respectively) are critical to anyone concerned with dieting. They increase fatty acid oxidation (burning of fat), basal metabolic rates and lower cholesterol. Omega-3 fatty acids also provide an anabolic effect by increasing the binding of IGF-1 to skeletal muscle and improving insulin sensitivity, even on diets high in fat which have a tendency to decrease insulin sensitivity.[47] As well, fish oils may also have important implications for women prone to osteoporosis since they appear to decrease calcium excretion.[48]

Omega-3's also stimulate prostaglandin production. Prostaglandins are eicosanoids that regulate activity in body cells on a moment-to-moment basis and are involved in critical functions like blood pressure regulation, insulin sensitivity, immune system and anti-inflammatory responses. They are also involved in literally hundreds of other functions, many of which have yet to be fully identified in research. If you have a problem producing prostaglandins or experience an imbalance between the different kinds of prostaglandins, overall health can be radically affected.

The series three prostaglandins are formed from EPA. As well, EPA reduces the production of the bad prostaglandins from arachidonic acid. EFA deficiency can lead to high blood pressure, hormonal dysfunction, impaired immune function, coagulation problems, inflammatory changes, dry itchy skin, peripheral edema and many other conditions.

Conjugated Linoleic Acid

Conjugated linoleic acid (CLA) is a mixture of isomers of linoleic acid, which is found preferentially in dairy products, meat, and in cheese, milks and yogurt that have undergone heat treatment. Supplementation with four ounces of cheddar cheese daily was found to increase the ratio of CLA to LA by 130%.

CLA has been shown to have properties above and beyond those of linoleic acid. It has shown potential as a powerful anticarcinogen[49,50] and has potent antioxidant activity.[51] Recent studies have suggested that CLA may be toxic to human cancer cells in the body.[52] Of the vast number of naturally occurring substances that have been demonstrated to have anticarcinogenic activity in experimental models, all but a handful of them are of plant origin. CLA is unique because it is present in food from animal sources, and its anticancer efficacy is expressed at concentrations close to human consumption levels.

So now we have a better understanding of the types of dietary fats and their influence on health. We can now discuss the importance of EFAs in the Metabolic Diet.

Essential Fatty Acids And The Metabolic Diet

EFAs can be beneficial even if a deficiency doesn't exist and, if used properly, can increase overall health, help you avoid heart disease and lose bodyfat. Overall, the increased processing of foods in our society has lowered the amount of EFAs in the average diet significantly. Foods rich in EFAs are highly perishable and not deemed practical or profitable for most commercial preparations. The extra EFAs you will get from the Metabolic Diet, as explained below, is just one more reason for giving the diet a try.

Earlier in this book we talked briefly about the omega-3's as a positive factor in high-fat diets. They are found to a high degree in fish oils (as EPA and DHA) and have been hailed as a major factor in lowering serum cholesterol levels, preventing coronary heart disease[53,54] and perhaps even preventing or curing atherosclerosis.[55]

Marine oils are a big part of the diets of Eskimo tribes. Though their higher-fat diet would seem to make them prime candidates for heart disease and atherosclerosis, they have been found to be almost immune to cardiovascular problems, at least until Western dietary influences in recent years. Studies have centered on omega-3 fatty acids in the fish oils and their cardioprotective capacities as being central to this phenomenon.[56]

For the person on the Metabolic Diet, where fat and protein are found at high levels, the omega-3's can provide an excellent hedge against worries about cholesterol. Blood pressure, clotting, immune response, insulin resistance and triglyceride levels are all positively affected.[57] Even in cases where dietary cholesterol is increased, omega-3's may aid in actually lowering serum cholesterol.[58] There is some evidence to suggest that in higher-fat diets aerobic exercise also reduces serum cholesterol[59] and thus may improve the effects of omega-3 rich fish oil on cholesterol.

LNA, EPA and DHA can also enhance lipolysis (bodyfat breakdown)[60,61] and decrease lipogenesis (bodyfat formation).[62,63] The combined breakdown of stored bodyfat and decrease in additional bodyfat can have very positive results for the dieter. You actually end up making less fat and breaking down more of what's already on the body when using these oils. EPA also decreases some of the possible inflammatory effects of using GLA supplements. That is because GLA can be a precursor for AA and the addition of EPA reduces DGLA conversion to AA, thus reducing AA accumulation in some cells and tissues secondary to GLA supplementation.[64]

That is why I wholeheartedly support adding portions of fish and fish oil to your daily diet. And, while many foods contain more than one type of fatty acid, plant oils are usually richer in unsaturated fatty acid content than animal fat. It's not surprising, then, that flaxseed oil, nuts, seeds and unprocessed vegetable oil are also rich in essential fatty acids.

That is also why I formulated an advanced EFA formula that contains all the "usual suspects" as well as other important ingredients. EFA+ is a multi purpose formulation designed to provide the full gamut of all the essential fatty acids that are so important in optimizing your metabolism, maximizing the anabolic and fat burning effects of exercise and decreasing the counter productive inflammatory response of exercise.

Fats and The Immune System

Besides the beneficial effects we have already discussed, fats can have dramatic effects on the immune system and can be used to treat patients with immune system problems. For example, it is known that the human immunodeficiency virus (HIV), is able to replicate in many human cells such as helper lymphocytes, monocytes/macrophages and glial cells. Monocytes/macrophages must be considered an important reservoir of HIV in the body and producers of cytokines such as interleukin-1 (IL1) and tumor necrosis factor (TNF).

These substances lead to a feedback loop that produces increased virus replication and a secondary production of other cytokines such as interleukin 6 (IL6) and granulocyte-macrophage colony stimulating factor (GM-CSF). These cytokines all together may be responsible for many clinical aspects of the HIV such as headache, fever, anorexia, subtle cognitive changes, and motor dysfunctions.

Omega 3 polyunsaturated fatty acids (omega 3-PUFA) are one of several compounds that can be used to both strengthen the host and attack the virus. Omegas 3-PUFAs have been shown to have significant modulating effects on the immune system in both man[65] and animals.[66] Their ability to decrease IL1 and TNF production by monocytes/macrophages and consequently of IL6 and several proteins may have beneficial effects on many clinical manifestations of AIDS.[67]

In the literature there are many confusing associations of dietary fat and immune function. It's well known that low fat diets suppress the immune system partly because of the potentially low levels of dietary essential fatty acids. Conversely, a recent study has shown that high fat intakes do not have any deleterious effects on the immune system of the well-trained runners.

In fact, a new study shows those athletes who train hard and cut back on fat may actually increase their susceptibility to infections and inflammation. Researchers found that long-distance runners who severely restricted their fat intake ended up depressing their immune systems. Runners who ate medium and high-fat diets (composed of 32 and 41 percent fat, respectively) had no immune system problems. Protein was kept at 15 percent no matter which diet the runners were on. An increase or decrease of carbohydrates made up the difference in calories between high and low-fat diets.

The higher-fat diets may lower proinflammatory cytokines, free radicals and hormones and enhance the levels of anti-inflammatory cytokines. Cytokines are messenger molecules that call cells to start or end inflammation at a site in the body. The inflammatory process is the body's response to infection or injury; swelling and pain can result as this tissue-repairing process takes place.

While researchers have shown that moderate exercise appears to enhance the immune system, very high intensity exercise has a negative effect on the immune system. A study investigating the effects of training intensity on the immune system used marathon runners because this sport tends to cause overtraining. As was revealed, the incidence of lingering upper respiratory infections was high in these athletes. I point this out because many athletes who train for a contest, especially bodybuilders and athletes competing in sports with weight classes, will select a low fat diet and tend to overtrain in this period. A moderate-fat diet would be a better choice as far as decreasing immune depression.

Bad Fats

There is a very popular misconception that commercial vegetable oils are a good healthy source for essential and non-essential fatty acids. Nothing could be farther from the truth. The fact is that most of those vegetable oils you see on the shelf of your local supermarket including corn, canola and soybean oils, have been hydrogenated or very heavily refined, and are so overly processed that they can be harmful to your health. Processing not only removes any useful properties the oil had such as EFAs or antioxidants, but depending on the processing can cause immune problems and predispose us to certain cancers.

The problem is that the natural poly- and monounsaturated fatty acids are reactive to light and heat and spoil readily. Even natural polyunsaturated fats, because they are unstable and oxidize readily, have been recently shown to have two serious drawbacks. First of all, they seem to promote certain cancers at a dietary concentration of 5% or more.[68] Secondly, while they can lower total cholesterol they can also lower the HDL[69] and thus increase the chances of coronary artery disease.

To make matters worse, polyunsaturated fats are usually treated in an effort to solve some of the problems associated with their commercial use. A process called hydrogenation has been used for decades to change natural oils into fats that are more solid and stable at room temperature, have a longer shelf life and are easier to use in certain foods and baked goods. Hydrogenation involves heating the oil in a vacuum and then forcing hydrogen through it under pressure. The process is continued until the required degree of hydrogenation is achieved.

Unfortunately, while hydrogenation and other methods used to refine or change oils, such as chemical solvents, bleaches and heat, may be healthy for business it isn't for our bodies. Not only do these processes destroy any natural qualities present in the natural oils, they create by-products that can be harmful to our health. Trans fatty acids, crosslinked fatty acid chains, and fragments of fatty acid chains produced secondary to hydrogenation can have significant adverse effects on blood cholesterol, increase the risk of heart disease. By competing with EFAs these fats lead to EFA deficiencies and subsequently to a host of other health problems including diabetes, cancer and weight gain.

Trans fatty acids have been the most widely researched of these toxic by-products. Trans fatty acids are found in refined vegetable oils, shortenings, almost all margarines and other oil-based foods, and even in baked and prepared snack foods such as cookies, crackers, and chips. Large quantities of unnatural trans fatty acids are also found as food contaminants during excessive heating of cooking oils for deep-frying and other excessive heat-requiring mass food preparation procedures. They have been found to raise overall cholesterol levels, lower HDL, decrease testosterone and insulin response, adversely affect liver enzyme activity and impair the immune system. They have thus been linked to heart disease, cancer and other diseases associated with aging.

Much of the problem resides with the fact that the shape of a fatty acid is essential to its proper functioning. While trans fatty acids have the same exact number of carbon and hydrogen atoms as the original fatty acid (known as the "cis-fatty acid"), its shape has been greatly changed. This change in shape, from "cis" fatty acid to "trans", causes competition for existing enzymes. As a result, the cis-fatty acids are unable to carry out their proper biological role.

The amount of trans fatty acids, or other toxic by-products, found in a food varies according to the extent and nature of the processing. Generally, vegetable oil products that are hard at room temperature (like shortening or margarine) are more riddled with trans fatty acids than products that are liquid at room temperature (like vegetable oil).

Recently, several studies have pointed to the adverse health effects of hydrogenated fats and the trans fatty acids in them (especially hard margarines, but even soft margarines are suspect), including an increased incidence of heart problems[70] likely secondary to unfavorable changes in serum lipoprotein[a], a strong risk factor for coronary heart disease.[71]

In addition to the well-recognized roles of EPA, the lack of trans fatty acids in the traditional Eskimo staple diet may also be responsible for their cardiovascular health. This diet contains cis-forms of the unsaturated fatty acids in physiologically optimal concentrations and is virtually totally devoid of unnatural and potentially hazardous trans and cis isomers of these fatty acids.[72] These differences in the Eskimo diet would likely ensure the synthesis of eicosanoids from dihomo-gamma-linolenic acid, arachidonic acid and eicosapentaenoic acid in balanced, optimal physiological concentrations.

Fats to Avoid

- All Margarines except those with low trans fatty acid content.
- Hydrogenated and Partially Hydrogenated Oil Products & Foods (check the labels)
- Shortening
- Old Fats and Oils Of Any Type

In summary, bad fats are fats that have been altered by processing and so that they compete with essential fatty acids and thus negatively affect cellular metabolism and structure. There is also some speculation that trans fatty acids may adversely affect insulin sensitivity, decrease fat oxidation and increase fat synthesis. All three of these effects would be counterproductive to anyone on the Metabolic Diet.

Foods containing significant amounts of trans fatty acids usually list hydrogenated or partially hydrogenated products in their listing of ingredients. These foods include baked goods, crackers, candies, almost all fried fast foods, potato chips, and other foods that have or are made with shortening, margarine or refined oils. Keep away from them as much as possible and use the fats recommended below.

GOOD & BAD FATS: USING YOUR HEAD

- Good Fats – EFAs, Fish oil, flax seed oil, GLA (EPO), Olive oil, some saturated fats.
- Bad Fats – too much saturated fats, trans fatty acids, MCTs.
- Fat content of foods can be changed. Examples are omega 3 enrichment of eggs by feeding flax seed to laying chickens. Also beef and pork meat fatty acid content can be manipulated.

Flaxseed Oil

Of the EFAs imbalances, LNA has created the most problems. Linoleic acid deficiency occurs much less frequently than LNA. Thus the diets of most people are much higher in LA than LNA. The excess LA seems to affect the biological action of LNA creating an even greater relative deficiency of LNA. With LNA and the other omega-3's responsible for most of the health benefits of EFAs listed above, this condition becomes even more serious.

One of the best-known sources of LNA (and a good source of LA) available is flaxseed oil (also known as flax oil or linseed oil). Hemp oil, another rich source of LNA (and LA and to a lesser extent GLA) is slowly becoming more available. Flaxseed oil consists of 45-65 percent LNA, 15 percent LA and a lesser amount of monounsaturated and saturated fatty acids.

Flaxseed oil can be an excellent source of LNA and I wholeheartedly support the addition of some flaxseed oil to any diet and, especially, the Metabolic Diet. However, there are some conflicting pieces of information that may limit the usefulness of flaxseed oil.

For example a recent study has shown that increasing dietary LNA (such as with the use of flaxseed oil) elevate tissue EPA concentrations in a predictable manner.[73] Now, we know that increased levels of EPA decrease the production of arachidonic acid and its metabolism into bad eicosanoids.[74] However, increased levels of LNA also decrease the production of GLA from LA because it inhibits the delta-6-desaturase enzyme that converts LA to GLA, and thus decreases the formation of certain good prostaglandins.

What can be we conclude from all this? Well, it seems that while flaxseed oil is a good supplement to our diets, it shouldn't be overdone. Enough should be used to increase our natural production of EPA but not to decrease the formation of GLA from LA. Thus, as well as some flaxseed oil, I recommend the use of GLA and EPA, as detailed below.

If you use flaxseed oil then make sure it's fresh. Flaxseed oil, like other perishable foods, will spoil or go rancid very quickly. That is why it needs to be refrigerated and used soon after opening. Look in any good health food store or nutritional center and you will find flaxseed oil in the refrigerated section. If you keep it refrigerated, flaxseed oil will generally last up to six weeks after it is opened.

I usually recommend a minimum of 5 grams of flaxseed oil per day to ensure you get the necessary EFAs. As well as the liquid form, flaxseed oil capsules are available and generally come in doses of 1 gram per capsule. Thus, you can use up to five capsules per day if no other flaxseed oil is used. Fresh unrefined flaxseed oil can also be added to a protein drink or salad (1-3 tablespoons) as a tasty way to supplement LNA.

Evening Primrose Oil And Borage Seed Oil

Both oils are rich in linoleic acid, vitamin E and GLA. Since GLA is a precursor for DGLA, which has been shown to be depleted by steroids, alcohol and other drugs, it has been suggested that GLA therefore provides protection for the liver. DGLA is easily produced from GLA and the use of GLA supplements may lead to the increased production of the good prostaglandins that help fight musculoskeletal inflammation, decrease cholesterol and fluid retention, and have beneficial effects on several hormones in the body.

Thus GLA may be helpful for several reasons. Evening primrose oil, for example, has been used as treatment for a variety of problems including PMS, chronic fatigue syndrome and arthritis. Since GLA is important for the production of several prostaglandins used to fight inflammation and muscle soreness in the body, it may be of great use to those involved in an advanced exercise program. If you suffer from any of these conditions you might want to give either oil a try.

In any case, for most of us, it's not a bad idea to supplement our diets with GLA. I usually recommend at least 500 mg of GLA daily. That usually translates to six or more capsules of evening primrose oil or three or more capsules of borage seed oil daily (evening primrose oil usually contains just less than half the amount of GLA as borage seed oil).

Fish And Fish Oils

Fish oils belong to the alpha-linolenic omega-3 series of fatty acids and are rich in eicosapentaenoic acid (EPA) as described above. While the body is able to convert alpha-linolenic acid to the longer chained EPA and DHA, it does so slowly. It makes good health sense to use fish oils since they are rich sources of EPA and DHA.

While increasing fat burning capabilities and lessening the amount of fat on the body, fish oils will also aid in limiting the breakdown of muscle tissue and adding muscle tone for increased body shaping. One of the ways that they do that is by increasing insulin sensitivity or on decreasing insulin resistance especially on high fat diets.[75]

They may also aid in lowering blood cholesterol levels, have vasodilatory effects (widening of the blood vessels), and may be protective[76] and perhaps even therapeutic[77] against certain cancers. EPA also seems to decrease the production of arachidonic acid (AA) from DGLA thus decreasing the production of some of the bad prostaglandins.

Fish oil also seems to have significant anti-inflammatory effects and protective effects on joint cartilage especially in arthritic conditions.[78] EPA and DHA seem to have some similar and independent effects on the body. For example, a recent study has found that DHA, rather than EPA is responsible for the anti-inflammatory effects of fish oil.[79]

The best way to obtain fish oil and thus your complement of these very important omega-3's is to regularly eat fresh fatty fish. For example, 100 grams (3.5 ounces) of Atlantic salmon has about 1400 milligrams of omega-3 fatty acids (EPA and DHA). Thus a half-pound of Atlantic salmon will give you an excellent daily complement of omega-3's (equal to or more than 10 capsules of fish oil).

Any fish – be it shell, freshwater, ocean or whatever – contains some omega-3 fatty acids. There is evidence, though, that ocean fish is a better source than freshwater fish (except for lake trout) for omega-3's. Fish from the colder northern waters such as the North Atlantic is superior to that caught near the Equator, and shellfish have lesser amounts of the omega-3's than other fish. Of the commonly available fish, the ones that are highest in omega-3's are salmon, herring, sardines, mackerel, and bluefish. I usually recommend that one or all of these fish be eaten at least three to four times a week.

On the other hand, there is no need to jump overboard on fish or fish oil consumption. In one study, researchers observed no significant associations between higher dietary intakes of fish, or the omega-3 fatty acids fish contained, and the risk of coronary artery disease (CAD).[80] Although men who never ate fish seemed to have a slightly higher risk of CAD than men who ate a small amount, increasing fish intake from one to two servings per week to five to six servings per week did not substantially reduce the risk of CAD among men who are initially free of cardiovascular disease.

Although further studies will have to be done to see if the results of this and other studies are valid, a recent review concluded that fish oil likely has beneficial effects on coronary artery disease and myocardial infarction.[81] On the basis of the many studies showing the benefits of fish oil, I recommend that fish or fish oil be used every day if possible or, if not, at least every other day.

If you have problems with eating fish on a regular basis, then I recommend that you use a fish oil supplement such as salmon oil capsules. Generally, I recommend 2,000 milligrams of EPA a day. Fish oil usually contains 20 percent EPA and a lesser amount of DHA so 10 capsules a day of 1,000 milligrams of fish oil should give you the recommended amount. If desired, or if there is a personal or family history of CAD, more fish oil could be consumed, as there appears to be no adverse metabolic effects of long-term fish oil supplementation.[82]

Whatever the amount that you use, be careful to buy fresh fish oil capsules that are in an opaque container. If the capsules are fishy tasting, chances are they are partially rancid and shouldn't be used. Keep the fish oil capsules in the refrigerator and away from light and use them up as soon as possible, at least within a few months of purchase.

Monounsaturated Fats

Monounsaturated fatty acids (oleic acid is the main one that concerns us), are produced by the body and are found in fats of both plant and animal origin. Animal sources of oleic acid are usually found along with saturated fatty acids and include beef, pork, lamb, chicken, turkey, dairy products, eggs, and some fish (like eel and trout). Although the common belief that the fats found in the above foods is all saturated fats, this is not the case. Oleic acid makes up from 20 to 50% of the fats in these foods.

The plant sources include olive, canola (rapeseed), hazelnut, and peanut oils as well as the foods from which these oils are extracted and also almonds, avocados, pistachios, and macadamia nuts. As well many of the foods that contain or are cooked in the above oils have significant levels of oleic acid. This includes fried foods, salad dressings, baked goods and certain soups.

Monounsaturated fatty acids, especially oleic acid, seem to have some advantages over other fatty acids. A significant intake of monounsaturated fatty acids will not increase your risk of heart disease and may even decrease it by their effects on total cholesterol, HDL and LDL.[83] The body also seems to have an easier time metabolically handling oleic acid over the other monounsaturated fatty acids.

Canola oil contains erucic acid that may have some toxic effects. As well, because of its method of extraction, canola oil contains some deformed fatty acids. Studies have also shown that, unlike olive oil use that can decrease total cholesterol and LDL, canola oil has no such effect on blood cholesterol[84].

For various reasons, olive oil seems to be one of the better fats to consume on the Metabolic Diet. But only certain olive oils are candidates. Like any other oil, any heat, chemical, solvents and other refining process ruins the health effect of olive oil. The best olive oil is the cold-pressed extra virgin olive oils since these oils are extracted by the use of gentle pressure rather than with the use of heat and solvents.

There is a body of epidemiological evidence that points to the health effects of olive oil.[85,86] As well, studies have shown that olive oil decreases atherogenesis.[87] Olive oil seems to one of the players responsible for the health effects of the Mediterranean Diet,[88] perhaps partly because of the antioxidant effect of the absorbable phenols that are present in olive oil.[8990] Additionally, very few pesticides and chemicals are needed to grow olives; therefore, you then have a source of fat that seems to have everything going for it. Olive oil is definitely a useful and necessary part of the Metabolic Diet.

Saturated Fats

Many of the foods recommended in the Metabolic Diet, such as red meat, eggs and cheese and butter contain saturated fats. These fats do have a tendency to raise total serum cholesterol and LDL levels in some individuals, especially those with previous blood cholesterol problems. The increase in total cholesterol is mainly from an increase in LDL although there is also a small increase in HDL.[91]

However, not all saturated fatty acids have an adverse effect on total cholesterol. For example, stearic acid (the main saturated fatty acid found in beef) and medium chain saturated fatty acids have little or no effect on total cholesterol. Recent studies have shown that replacement of carbohydrates with stearic acid (as is done to some extent in the high-fat, low-carb phase of the Metabolic Diet) has little effect on lipid and lipoprotein concentrations in plasma.[92,93] As well, in these studies oleic and linoleic acids had beneficial effects on blood lipids by raising HDL and lowering LDL.

It's important to realize that recent research has shown that it is the oxidized forms of cholesterol and LDL that increase the incidence of cardiovascular disease (CVD) including CAD.[94] Thus, factors that decrease the tendency of LDL to oxidize (such as the use of monosaturated and marine oils) can negate any harmful effects a higher-fat diet may have on CVD.

As well, natural saturated fats do not have the toxic harmful effects seen with the use of trans fatty acids. They are mainly an effective and compact source of energy. Most of us have no real problem with these saturated fats – our bodies know how to deal with them.

Saturated fats are an integral part of the Metabolic Diet. If used properly, natural saturated fats will help you to lose weight and bodyfat. Any adverse effects that they might have on those susceptible to cholesterol problems are usually diminished by the fact that the dietary as well as the body's saturated fats are used as a primary source of energy, and therefore do not have a chance to do any harm. As well, other recommended fats can decrease or eliminate any adverse changes of the Metabolic Diet to total cholesterol, HDL and LDL.

Butter Or Margarine?

Lately the marketing of low trans fatty acid margarines has confused the issue of whether you should use margarine or butter, or neither. At the heart of this debate is trans fatty acids, a type of fat found in margarine and many processed and fast foods. At one time, trans fatty acids were thought to be better for you than saturated fat in butter. But some studies have found that trans fatty acids may be harmful to your health as saturated fat and possibly worse. So does this mean you should switch back to butter? Most health experts say no. But they do recommend limiting trans fat in your diet.

But when you want to use butter or margarine, which is better? Most health experts say margarine, particularly the tub and squeeze-bottle kinds, which are more liquid. They usually contain less trans fat than do stick margarines. In addition, some manufacturers have developed margarine spreads and sticks that contain no trans fat. As is often the case, the key is moderation.

How Much And What Kind Of Fats Do We Eat?

In a diet where fat plays the key role as it does in the Metabolic Diet, it's important to get a handle on just what kind of fats you should be looking for and in what proportion they should be eaten. Taking into consideration everything we have just said about fats, the following guidelines will make the Metabolic Diet healthier and more effective.

BE WISE WITH FATS

- Eat fewer processed baked goods and fried foods, especially fast foods.
- Bake, boil, microwave, poach or steam foods instead of frying them.
- Buy oils that are predominantly monounsaturated (olive or canola oils).
- Consume only fresh oils.

Twenty-five percent of your fat intake should come from olive oil and the EFA-rich foods mentioned above. These include nuts, seeds, fish, flaxseed oil, salmon oil, and unprocessed vegetable oils. The other 75 percent of your fat intake should come from high quality meats, chicken, eggs, cheese, pork, butter, shell and other fish and associated foods. Also, make an effort to use the omega-3 enriched eggs and dairy products. Table I provides an easy way to judge the various fats in some common foods and oils.

You should do your best to avoid the "bad fats" listed previously. Margarine (because of its trans fatty acid content) and commercial processed vegetable oils are a no-no. Hydrogenated oil products and shortening, which are found in almost every processed food, should also be avoided.

In fact, any kind of oil that has been around for a while should be suspect, even fish oils. If they have been stored too long, there is a good chance they have oxidized to some extent and can cause free radical damage in the body. As well, they likely contain altered fatty acid derivatives that are harmful to your health.

You should supplement your diet with GLA-containing oils (such as evening primrose or borage seed oils), unspoiled fish oil (if your intake of fish is lacking) and to a lesser extent flaxseed oils as discussed previously. You should make liberal use of extra virgin olive oil for preparing foods, salads, protein drinks and in any other way that you find palatable.

Fatty Acid Composition Of Commonly Consumed Foods
(as percentage of total fatty acids)

Food	Saturated	Monounsaturated	Polyunsaturated
Butter, Cream, Milk	65	30	05
Beef	46	48	06
Bacon and pork	38	50	12
Lard	42	45	13
Chicken	33	39	28
Fish	29	31	40
Coconut oil	92	06	02
Palm kernel oil	86	12	02
Cocoa butter	63	34	03
Olive oil	15	76	09
Peanut oil	20	48	32
Cottonseed oil	27	20	53
Soybean oil	16	24	60
Corn oil	13	26	61
Sunflower seed oil	11	22	67
Safflower seed oil	10	13	77

Reading Between The Lines On Labels

How can you tell if a food product contains trans fat? When it comes to listing fat on food labels, manufacturers are required to only list total fat and saturated fat. Some also voluntarily list monounsaturated and polyunsaturated fat, but it's unlikely you will see trans fat listed. Still, you may be able to tell if a product contains trans fat, even if it's not directly listed on the food label.

Look for the words "hydrogenated" or "partially hydrogenated" in the list of ingredients. These terms indicate that the product contains trans fat. However, you will not be able to tell how much trans fat is included.

If you want to learn more about good fats and bad fats and the effects they can have on your health, then I recommend you read *Fats that Heal Fats that Kill* by Udo Erasmus, published by *alive* Books, 7436 Fraser Park Drive, Burnaby, BC, Canada, V5J 5B9. This book, while being almost encyclopedic in scope, is easy to read and understand.

CHAPTER SIX

Measuring Your Body Composition and Tracking Your Progress

The most accurate and scientific way to determine your bodyfat percentage is by hydrostatic weighing. This test is conducted in special tank and compares your weight completely under (with all air exhaled out of our lungs) and out of water. Hydrostatic weighing is based on the concept that the density and gravity of lean tissue is greater than that of fat tissue, so lean tissue will sink in water and fat tissue will float. While hydrostatic weighing is the best measurement, it can be costly, inconvenient and time-consuming. Other methods of determining bodyfat levels, such as the Bod Pod, a device that uses air displacement instead of water, while more convenient are also costly and unavailable to most of us.

Another way to measure bodyfat percentage is with anthropometric measurements. Measurements are taken with a measuring tape at sites where fat is usually distributed, such as the waist and thigh. Specific equations are used to calculate the bodyfat percentage. These measurements while less costly and easier to do but are not very accurate.

Overall, bodyfat percentage can best be measured with skin fold calipers. If done correctly calipers are an accurate, inexpensive and convenient way to measure the thickness of subcutaneous fat. This technique involves measuring fat levels in the body by assessing levels at certain key fat depots with the skin calipers. You can have the skin fold test performed by a professional, or you can do it yourself by purchasing the calipers, along with easy to follow instructions.

MEASURING YOUR PROGRESS

- Weight Can Be Misleading – depending on fluid retention in the short term and on changes in body composition in the long term.
- Someone may weigh the same but have much higher muscle mass and lower bodyfat.

With the calipers you can determine your percentage bodyfat by taking skin density measurements of the suprailliac area. This area is approximately one inch above the right hipbone about five inches or so to the right of and just below your belly button (see Figure x). As per the diagram, while standing firmly pinch the suprailliac skinfold between your left thumb and forefinger. Place the jaws of the calipers over the skinfold while continuing to hold the skinfold with the left hand. Then take your measurement as per the instructions and the diagram. Once you have the measurement refer to the bodyfat interpretation chart (included with the calipers) to determine your bodyfat percentage.

While knowing your bodyfat level is a step forward, it tells you nothing about your level of lean body mass. To get the complete picture and accurately measure your present status and progress we need to find out our Metabolic Index.

OTHER WAYS TO MEASURE PROGRESS

- Mirror.
- The way clothes fit.
- What people say.
- Body Mass Index – height and weight formula that can't take into account body composition.
- Measuring bodyfat is only a measure of fat loss.
- The Metabolic Index.

The Accu-Measure® Calipers

As I have already explained hydrostatic weighing is the best way to measure your bodyfat percentage. The most accurate of the easy to use alternatives are the skin fold calipers.

For the purposes of the Metabolic Diet and to keep things as simple as possible, we will only measure one site. The Accu-Measure® Calipers (available from **www.MetabolicDiet.com**) is a precision instrument which has been shown in comparative studies to be closer in accuracy to the "gold standard" underwater weighing than any of the more elaborate methods of measuring bodyfat (without the inconvenience, expense and trained personnel and lack of privacy that these other methods entail).

With the calipers you can determine your percentage bodyfat by taking skin density measurements of the suprailliac area. This area is approximately one inch above the right hipbone about five inches or so to the right of and just below your belly button (Figures 1- 5).

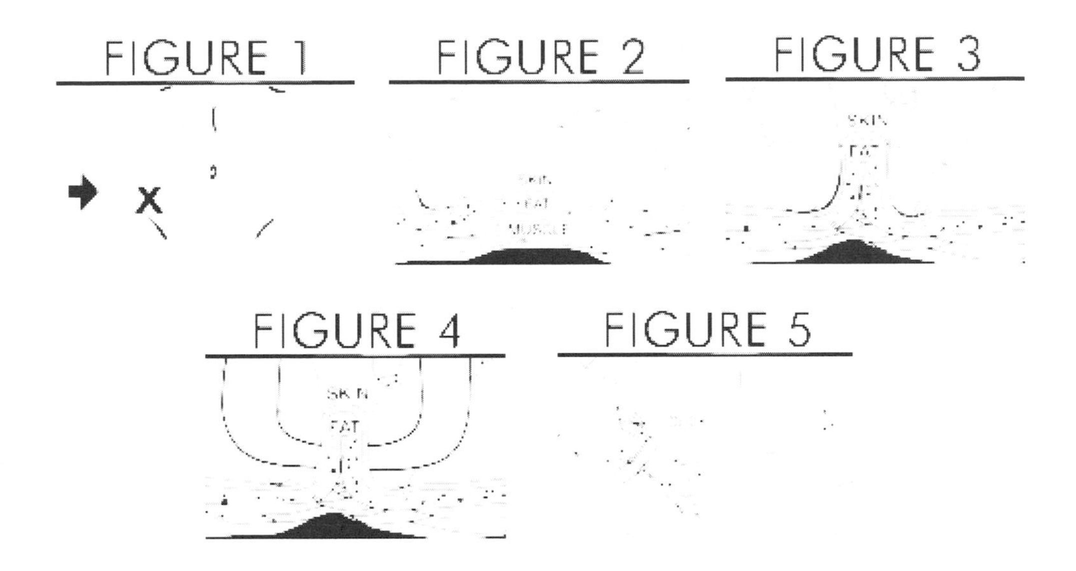

As per the diagram, while standing firmly pinch the suprailliac skinfold between your left thumb and forefinger. Place the jaws of the calipers over the skinfold while continuing to hold the skinfold with the left hand. Then take your measurement as per the instructions and the diagram. Once you have the measurement refer to the bodyfat interpretation chart below (also included with the calipers) to determine your bodyfat percentage.

While knowing your bodyfat level is a step forward, it tells you nothing about your level of lean body mass. To get the complete picture and accurately measure your present status and progress we need to use my Metabolic Index.

The Metabolic Index

The Metabolic Index (MIDx) is the best way to measure your progress while you are on the Metabolic Diet. The MIDx takes into account all the variables that other methods cannot. Not only does it address the height/weight issue but also the degree of bodyfat. With the MIDx you get a snap shot of your body composition and progress.

What is the MIDx and what does it measure? The MIDx is a ratio derived by considering not only weight and height but also your percentage of bodyfat. It uses a very easy formula for calculating. In fact, just fill in your weight in pounds, your height in inches and your bodyfat level as a percentage into the following formula and do the calculations.

FIGURING OUT THE MIDx

Body weight in pounds divided by the height in inches squared and the results multiplied by 7,250 and the results divided by the percent bodyfat.

➲ {(body weight in pounds) / (height in inches)^2 * 7,250} / % bodyfat.

Or if you are using the Metric system:

➲ {(body weight in kilograms) / (height in meters)^2 * 10.3} / % bodyfat.

In my case, using pounds and inches, my MIDx is 185 / (66)2 * 7,250 divided by 10%

(185 / 4356) * 7,250 / 10
MIDx = 30.8

An easier way to figure out your MIDx is to go to **http://www.metabolicdiet.com/index2.htm** and plug in your stats. Since it's so easy to do you can check your MIDx often and use it as a guide and measure of your progress.

The MIDx is much more advanced than the commonly used and accepted body mass index (BMI). The trouble with the BMI is it cannot tell if you are overweight because you are fat or if you are heavier than they figure you should be because you have got more muscle mass than the average couch potato.

For example, even though I am heavy for my height, I have a fair amount of muscle mass and a low bodyfat. So rather than looking fat I look trim and muscular. A couch potato with the same height and weight would definitely be fat. The big difference, besides the obvious aesthetics, is that while the couch potato has to carry his fat, my muscle carries me.

If I use the MIDx, not only do I get a more realistic look at my body composition, but I can also track my progress to improving even further. Let us say that I go on the Metabolic Diet and get down to a minimal 175 lbs and 8% bodyfat. My MIDx would then be 36. The increase in the MIDx shows that at 175 lbs. and 8 % bodyfat I am carrying less fat in proportion to my muscle mass than at 185 lbs. and 10% bodyfat. If you was able to increase lean body mass while losing bodyfat to the point of maintaining my weight, then the MIDx would increase even more. At 185 lbs and 8% bodyfat my MIDx would be 38.5. When the MIDx increases, regardless of the starting point, it shows that you are making progress because you are increasing the ratio between muscle mass and bodyfat by decreasing bodyfat and/or increasing muscle mass.

The important thing about the MIDx is that it will give you a starting point and from there an indication of how you are progressing every step of the way. Once you have established your baseline MIDx it's easy to objectively see if you are making progress, if you are losing bodyfat but not at the expense of important muscle mass. If the MIDx is going up, even minimally, you are making progress.

The higher the Metabolic Index, up to a point, the better your improvement and the closer you are to your goals. The lower the Metabolic Index is, the more room for improvement there is and a determination of just how much more you have to go to reach your goals.

The ideal for the average woman is different than the ideal for average man. For women the ideal is around 13 to 20 while for men it's between 22 to 32. In reality the final point doesn't really matter since it's the improvement that counts. As long as the index keeps going up then there is some improvement being made. Once the index gets above 18 for women and 32 for men you have looking at muscle mass and bodyfat levels that are too extreme for many people but not to those who aspire to bodybuilding and competitive fitness standards. Competitive bodybuilders will be looking to get their MIDx well over 40. Olympia level bodybuilders will have a MIDx over the 100 mark.

In reality, the MIDx is an indicator that when you are losing weight you are close to maintaining or even increasing lean body mass as you lose bodyfat. In fact, the more lean body mass you have and the less fat the better the index. If someone loses even a lot of weight but loses too much lean body mass the index will not improve all that much. What that means is that even though the person has lost weight they look very flabby and therefore lost the weight by sacrificing muscle mass. This is exactly the opposite of what most people want.

Now that you have determined our Metabolic Index and we know how to measure our muscle mass, weight and fat loss progress, you can go ahead and set your weight/muscle mass/fat loss goals.

THE METABOLIC INDEX™

The **Metabolic Index** (MIDx) is the best way to measure your progress while you're on The Metabolic Diet. The MIDx takes into account all the variables that other methods can't. Not only does it address the height/weight issue but also the degree of bodyfat. With the MIDx you get a snap shot of your body composition and progress.

The MIDx is a ratio derived by considering not only weight and height but your percentage of bodyfat. Just plug your information into formula, in Metric or English.

CHAPTER SEVEN

Periodizing the Metabolic Diet and Metabolic Diet Supplements

The Metabolic Diet will work for anyone who wants to lose weight and bodyfat while at the same time maintain or gain muscle mass. That includes those who are just interested in looking fit and toned to the bodybuilder who wants to get into competitive shape.

This section of the Anabolic Solution includes specific information for anyone looking to gain muscle mass and lose bodyfat, including recreational and competitive bodybuilders, on how to use the Metabolic Diet in the best way possible to get the results they want.

We will discuss how to use the Metabolic Diet in different phases of their bodybuilding training and competition, and how and when to use some appropriate nutritional supplements for the fastest results. The starting point will be the Strict Phase of the Metabolic Diet. Carbs can be increased if need be after three to four weeks.

In this section I will give you some points for calculating starting calories for the various training and pre-competitive phases. These values are not written in stone and serve only as starting points for your journey of self-discovery. Depending on your metabolism and situation, you will have to experiment to find what is optimal for you.

Diet Phases

There are five phases of the diet where adjustments will be made based on progress toward a competition. The mass, cutting and pre-contest phases will be familiar to most bodybuilders. We also include a Start-Up Phase in our diet plan. Just as the training volume and intensity in bodybuilding must be phase specific, taking into account the scope of training for each particular phase, so must the diet and nutritional supplements use.

A good bodybuilding program is one that improves muscle size, tone, density, and definition. A training program is successful only when it has these characteristics:

- It is a part of a longer plan.
- It is based on the scientific knowledge available in the field.
- It uses **Periodization** as a guideline for planning training throughout the year.

The program must have short-term goals and long-term goals that are phase specific. Each training phase has its own objectives, so it is necessary to adapt the diet and supplements to the goals of each phase and to coincide with the overall plan.

The compilation of a plan with both short- and long-term goals must take into account the individual's background, physical potential, and rate of adaptation to the physiological challenges imposed by training.

Using The Metabolic Diet and Supplements in the Different Training Phases

In my view there are only four basic training phases that are needed to reach your goal as far as body composition, bodybuilding or strength, with a fifth phase added for competitive bodybuilders. The goal in all cases, is to increase lean body mass and decrease bodyfat to some degree or another. The competitive bodybuilder is at one end of the scale while the person who just wants a fit and toned body is on the other. While the goals may be different the path is the same. It's all just a matter of degree.

Some people add a rest phase, particularly after a competition. In this phase you basically chill out, eat, drink and be merry. Usually a few weeks is more than enough to regain some sort of physical and psychological balance after a grueling and stressful competition. Once you are rested a few weeks, or more, you start back into the Start-Up Phase.

1. **Start-Up Phase**
2. **Mass Phase**
3. **Strength Phase**
4. **Cutting Phase**
5. **Pre-competition Phase**
6. **Rest Phase**

For maximum results you will have to use some nutritional supplements to complement the various phases of training and the diet. Like the training and diet, the intelligent cycling of your supplement use will allow you to get the best results possible. The supplements will enhance the anabolic effects of your training and the Metabolic Diet. Detailed information on each of the supplements is available in Appendix One.

This is Not a Training Book

It's important to realize that I have no aspirations about giving you comprehensive powerlifting and training information and routines. This is not a training book, but rather a nutrition book that shows you how to modify the Metabolic Diet and the use of my **MD+** line of nutritional supplements to your training routines, whatever they may be. How you train (whether you do one set to failure or a dozen), the exercises you do and the way that you do them, the number of workouts per day and week, the weights you use and how you use them,. is up to you.

But always keep an open mind and keep experimenting with both innovative and conservative approaches to training. You are never good enough so that you cannot improve even further.

Also keep in mind that although there are people who swear by their method of training, that doesn't mean it's the best one for you. It also doesn't mean it will not work for you. Sometimes it's not so much the training but the motivation and enthusiasm behind that training that pushes you to new heights. And as long as you do not get injured and you are making progress, then stick with it for as long as it works.

So while this isn't a training book, I will cover some of the basics and will also toss in my two cents worth anytime I feel like it. After all I have been weight training for almost 40 years, on a competitive level in powerlifting for more than half of that time, and I have learned a little along the way.

On the other hand if you want to delve more deeply into the world of bodybuilding, including training routines, articles, tips, editorials, what's popular, old time stuff, rants and takes on almost everything that involves bodybuilding, then go to **www.CoachSOS.com** and head over to the bodybuilding section. I will be developing this site over the next few months so you will have to be patient at first.

I am also planning to have some top notch bodybuilding coaches on hand to help you out and answer some of your questions, including a sections for information, news, articles, and contest results. Although both my primary sites, which also includes

www.MetabolicDiet.com, are up and running and contain a ton of information already, they will not be fully up and going until sometime near the end of 2002.

Training Basics

Although this is not a training book, some training basics are a prerequisite to using the diet and supplements to the best advantage and getting big and cut. As such I will glancingly cover some of the more common questions you might have and also a few odds and ends that I think are important if you want to train and compete effectively.

When you are setting up your weight training program, remember to include all the body parts, starting with the large muscle groups, working your way down to the smaller muscle groups.

How Much Weight Should You Use?

The easiest way to determine how much weight you should use, especially when you are first starting out or beginning a routine with exercises you are not familiar with, on each lift is to try a light weight for a warmup. If it's easy to do more than 10 reps then add some more weight and try it again. Continue doing this until you find a weight that taxes your abilities after as many reps as you are going to be doing.

At first, it's better to go too light than too heavy so it's best to find a weight that you find fairly easy to do for at least ten reps. In your next session, once your muscle soreness has improved and after a few warm up sets, try the same weight that you left off with for your first set. Then increase the weights for each set from there on until you find it difficult to do 12 reps (or 15 or whatever number of reps you have to do in each set). Then depending on your routine you may stay at that weight or increase the weight and decrease the reps and build up again to the number of reps you want to get.

How About the Number of Reps/Sets?

That all depends on your routine. It can vary from one set per exercise to several sets and from a few reps to a few dozen or more. The rule of thumb is that if you want to gain muscle mass and strength you should do more than one set or take that set and do as many reps as you can until exhausted (HIT principle).

How Long Should You Rest Between Exercises/Workout Sessions?

It all depends on your goals. If you are after strength and are using heavy weights (high intensity training) then you will need more rest between sets. That is because it takes longer for you to be mentally and physically ready to lift near maximum weights. If you are using lighter weights then 30 seconds to one minute is usually enough and may in fact be optimal to maximize muscle toning and decreasing bodyfat. In all cases it's usually a good idea to not train the same bodypart in consecutive days with a minimum of 48 hours of rest between training sessions.

Choosing Your Exercises

Choosing exercises can be the hardest part of your routine. Why? Because there are so many exercises out there, how do you know which ones to do? Which ones work the chest and which ones work the biceps? Should you watch other people at the gym and do what they are doing? In general, it's best not to do an exercise just because you see someone else doing it. That person may be an advanced exerciser and what they are doing could injure you. Also, how do you know they are doing it right?

One option for choosing exercises is to hire a personal trainer. A good personal trainer can help you figure out what to do and how to do it. If that is not an option, consider renting or buying a workout video. Strength training videos can give you a start by giving you visual instruction without the cost of a personal trainer.

Sequence of Exercises

Make sure you choose at least one exercise for each major muscle group. The muscles you want to work include: Chest, back, shoulders, biceps, triceps, quadriceps, hamstrings, calves and abdominals. If you leave any muscle group out, this could cause an imbalance in your muscles, result in an unbalanced physique and possibly lead to injuries.

The order in which you do your exercises is important. I usually recommend starting with your larger muscle groups and then training the smaller muscle groups. That is because working the large muscle groups takes more out of you and you do not need as much to work the small muscle groups. If you were to do the small muscle groups first you would not have the energy and stamina you need to work harder with the heavier weights.

Changing Training Routines

Now that you know the basic variables that go into a complete strength training routine, you can manipulate these variables at any point during your workout to constantly challenge your muscles. Most people will experience a weight loss/strength training plateau about 4 to 6 weeks after starting a new program. At that time you should change your program to include new exercises or variations of the same exercises.

What Warm-ups Should I Do? And What About Stretching?

I am not a big fan of stretching. I guess I got turned off by seeing those jokers with the broom sticks working out with the wood for 30 minutes before they did their max 135 lb squats. But there is more to it than that. Stretching too much, especially past the normal range of motion and/or when you are cold, will set you up for injuries. And frankly you do not need to stretch prior to lifting unless you are also into ballet.

I am also not a fan of doing any kind of extensive warmup prior to lifting. Two or three good warm-up sets before getting into the serious weights is all you really need. Do a couple of warm-up sets in the specific exercise you are doing before you get on with the heavier weights. The best way to do the first few sets is to feel it out, go to the limits of the lift, hold it there for a few seconds, make sure you are in the groove. The warm up sets give you the flexibility and balance you need to do the lift properly and allow you to get your neural mechanisms in gear so that you will be able to control and better handle the heavier weight.

For example in the squat, the first warm-up should be really light, maybe just the bar with a flywheel on each side (a 45 lb plate) for 10 slow deliberate reps. How many warm-ups you do depends on how much weight you intend to haul. For example if you are into a heavy duty strength routine and going for heavy triples and doubles you may need four and likely more sets before you are ready. For example if I intended to double 700 lbs, I'd start with 225 lbs (I never liked starting off with just one lonely plate a side) and do 8 to 10 reps. Then jump to 315 for six reps, 405 for 4 reps, 495 for three reps, 565 for three reps, 615 for three, 650 for a double, 675 for a double and finally 700 for a double. In this set of squats, the first four would be warm-ups, while the other five would be work sets. You can do it with all kinds of different jumps but you get the picture.

How many warm up sets should you do? There is no set number. You should warm up until you feel comfortable with the exercise and are solidly in your lifting groove. Depending on how you feel that day, it may take a few more warmup sets before you get into the proper frame of mind to make those heavy lifts, both in training and competition.

Warm-ups become even more important if you are trying to train with one or more minor injuries or when you are feeling really tight. In cases like these the warm-up will either get you ready to lift the heavy iron, or tell you to throw in the towel and work your forearm and calves instead.

What about some cooling down exercises after a heavy workout?

The best cool down exercise I found was trying to put my clothes back on and crawl out of the gym. On the other hand if you are going to do some aerobics, it's best to do it now rather than at the beginning of your workout. Better still, schedule your aerobics at another time.

What Supplements Should I Use?

I thought you'd never ask.

My MD+ Line of Targeted Nutritional Supplements

I formulated a complete nutritional supplement line, which includes over 25 cutting edge products designed to work with the Metabolic Diet and to maximize body composition, athletic performance and the beneficial effects of exercise. These formulations were done using the latest scientific and medical information, along with the knowledge and expertise I have accumulated in the last four decades. I have tried to use the best ingredients available regardless of costs to form products that are far superior to any on the market today.

Supplements that can be used in any phase of training, including the traditional Mass and Cutting Phases.

1. **MVM** – a comprehensive, specially balanced multiple vitamin and mineral formula designed to provide full-spectrum nutrition with an emphasis on the needs of athletes and anyone who exercises.

   → Provides protective properties against marginal deficiencies of vitamins and minerals.

   → Optimizes the effect of training.

   → Acts as the foundation for your body's nutritional needs.

2. **EFA+** – A complete essential and synergistic fatty acid formulation designed to provide the full gamut of all the essential fatty acids that are so important to optimizing your metabolism, maximizing the anabolic and fat-burning effects of exercise and dealing with minor muscle ache after exercise.

   Provides you with a specially balanced blend of the omega-3 and omega-6 essential fatty acids plus several other natural ingredients to optimize the anabolic and fat burning effects of exercise.

   The formulation acts to increase fatty acid oxidation, improve insulin sensitivity and serum cholesterol levels, aid in injury prevention and treatment, and support proper cardiovascular, nervous system function, and immune system function.

3. **Antiox** – complex and complete antioxidant formulation that provides targeted antioxidant support to all tissues in the body including the musculoskeletal system and the liver.

   Antiox contains the usual antioxidants beta-carotene, vitamins C and E, and it also contains immune enhancers including glutathione, the most important, all-purpose, endogenous antioxidant in our bodies. Our brand of glutathione is absorbed from the GI tract and used both systemically in all tissues in the body, but especially by the liver in its role as the primary detoxifying organ in the body. As well, Antiox contains other effective ingredients including lipoic acid, lycopene, resveratrol (from red wine) and grape seed extract.

- ➔ Increases natural muscle recovery from the effects of excessive exercise.
- ➔ Protects healthy tissues in the body.

4. **Regulate** – is an effective blend of natural soluble and insoluble fibers formulated to deal with occasional constipation and frequent bowel movements and keep the GI tract healthy. The various soluble fibers and other compounds contained in Regulate have also been found useful to:

    - ➔ Maintain cholesterol levels that are already within normal range;
    - ➔ Support a healthy heart
    - ➔ Increase natural insulin sensitivity.
    - ➔ Has probiotic effects – promotes growth of beneficial bacteria in bowels.

    As well, Regulate, by delaying gastric emptying and reducing the time to perceived fullness, is effective as an appetite suppressant. Taken before meals or whenever hungry, Regulate lessens your hunger and curbs cravings.

5. **Exersol** (combination of Resolve, Power Drink and Amino)– to maximize the anabolic and fat burning effects of exercise.

6. **MRP LoCarb** – An engineered high-protein, low-carbohydrate and moderate-fat meal replacement powder containing an advanced protein blend, healthy fats, and a balanced array of vitamins and minerals. It contains no trans fatty acids, only I gram of saturated fat, and only 5 grams of carbs per serving. Of those five grams of carbs, three are a combination of soluble and insoluble fiber, leaving only 4 grams of carbs that are absorbed.

7. **LoCarb Sports Bars** have the nutritional advantages of the MRP LoCarb meal replacement powders in a convenient and delicious bar. The bars can be used post-workout, or as a snack anytime since they can be easily kept nearby in your gym bag, desk drawer, purse, glove compartment etc.

    - ➔ Formulated to improve fatigue, prevent overtraining and to enhance the immune system. Also to normalize the metabolism and to naturally support thyroid, testosterone, GH, insulin and adrenergic function. It's the perfect nutritional supplement to deal with stress, fatigue and the overtraining syndrome.

8. **Joint Support** – With its many ingredients, Joint Support is useful in combating inflammation and preventing and treating injuries. By providing some of the raw materials that are essential for the body's natural synthesis and maintenance of joints, ligaments, muscles and tendons. Joint Support protects joints and other tissues from the effects of excessive exercise and overtraining.

We will discuss the supplements that can be used in more detail under the various training phases.

Start Up Phase

After a lay off or even when just starting out it's a mistake to get right into it. There is no place for any routine that immediately concentrates on increasing muscle mass or increasing definition. Both your body and mind have to be conditioned for the more specific phases that follow.

It's important to get your system ready for the stress and strain of the coming programs. In short you need to build a sturdy foundation on top of which you can lay on layers of sculpted muscle.

As such, the Start Up training should consist of some progressive circuit type training. At first one set after another of a number of different exercises, using a very light load for the first few sessions, is the way to go. You can gradually increase the weight and resistance but not to the point where you are ever going all out. As well, keep the repetitions in the 12 to 15 range all throughout this phase and the training time under one hour.

How long should you stay in this phase. It all depends on how long it's been since you trained and how burned out you are. Usually two to six weeks is enough with 4 weeks being about right.

ADAPTATION

- Adaptation to training and diet, making it as easy as possible, is the hallmark of the Start Up Phase.
- Keep weight constant – shift in body composition.
- Need high level of dietary fat in this phase.

Nutrition for the Start Up Phase

We will make the assumption that you are beginning the Metabolic Diet during this phase, although this may not necessarily be the case it makes the most sense.

During most of the Metabolic Diet, you will not find yourself restricting calories much. In fact, some people may find they have a problem getting enough, especially in the Mass Phase. Even in other phases, many will find that with increased training and exercise, they can take in a huge amount without suffering any consequences. The only phase that usually requires a gradual reduction in calories is the Cutting (definition) Phase.

At the beginning, though, we want to make the switch as easily as possible. That is why it's important not to jump right in at a low calorie level. Often the fatigue and discomfort you may feel is simply from a lack of food rather than a lack of carbs. And if some of is from the actual metabolic switch, it's compounded if you are starving. Also I do not want you feeling bloated and suffering too much from the constipation and/or diarrhea that you may have as a result of the sometimes radical change in your macronutrient intake. Dieting per se often affects the bowels and can compound any effect that may come from starting on the Metabolic Diet.

That is why your STARTING POINT FOR DAILY CALORIES ON THIS DIET SHOULD BE 18 TIMES YOUR BODYWEIGHT in pounds (or 40 times your bodyweight in Kg). If you are 200 pounds, this would call for 200 X 18 or 3,600 calories a day during the weekday portion of the diet. This makes for a "static" phase where you lose some bodyfat, gain some muscle mass and maintain about the same weight. This is a phase where you will be changing the ratio of internal masses to some degree but most of what you are trying to do is allow your body its easiest path toward adapting to the diet.

As you continue in this phase you should experiment with the formula above as a way of finding precisely where your "maintenance" level for calories is. This will let you know from what point you need to add or subtract calories for gains or losses in other parts of the diet. It's also not a bad idea to keep a 2-3 day diary of what you are eating and then have someone who has some expertise in diets look at it. That way you will get numbers and foods you can best work with and figure what you need precisely for maintenance.

You will need a fiber supplement when you first start the diet. One of the results of the Metabolic Diet is that the bowels must readjust to all that meat. The fats can act as a stool softener and you may experience some diarrhea. You will need to firm them up with some fiber. The radical change in diet can also cause constipation.

Most of the problems we have found with people initiating the diet fall in this area and their failure to take the fiber necessary to harden stools or push processed food through the eliminative tract. You may be able to get away with just eating bran but there is a good chance you will need a supplement to best get through this period.

But soluble and insoluble fiber has other purposes. Fiber has multiple effects on both the body and the GI tract, and is thought to be useful in the management and prevention of high cholesterol and triglycerides, prostate problems and diabetes. Fiber becomes even more important as you drop your calories since it decreases hunger and keeps the bowels in synch, as well as providing some antioxidant effects from the digestion of the soluble fibers by gut bacteria, all of which become more important as you drop calories and the amount of food you eat.

As far as the phase shift, increasing the fiber in the diet decreases the absorption rate of the weekend carbs and dampens the effects of high glucose/insulin levels, as well as providing the above benefits.

The nutritional supplement line I formulated for the Metabolic Diet includes **Regulate**, a multi-ingredient low-carb supplement (none of the fiber is absorbed) meant to regulate the bowels and keep the whole intestinal tract healthy. It's combination of ingredients, including several soluble and insoluble fibers, works like a charm.

If you use a commercial product such as Metamucil be careful of hidden carbohydrates. Often, refined carbs are used to make them taste better so check the carb count on the package before purchasing them.

You will probably have to take the fiber supplement for the first few weeks to a month of the diet, or for some for a few months. In most cases, by that time, your body will have fully adapted to it. If not, it's a good idea to stay on a fiber supplement on a regular or on an as needed basis.

Some bodybuilders have also found that taking a meal high in fiber, like a Caesar Salad, in the middle of the day will do the trick. This will provide about 7 1/2 grams of carbs and, as long as you stick close to overall carb limits, shouldn't present any problem. Especially after you have been on the diet for a while.

NUTRITION FOR THE START UP PHASE

- Begin first 12 days then weekend carb up then 5-6 days low carb and one to two days high carb.
- No change in calories, substitute fat and protein for carbs
- STARTING POINT FOR DAILY CALORIES ON THIS DIET SHOULD BE 18 TIMES YOUR BODYWEIGHT in pounds or 40 times your bodyweight in kg.

Watch For Hidden Carbs

The start up phase will run smoother and get you in gear quicker if you remember that refined carbs are hidden in almost everything you will find on those supermarket shelves. Seasoning, ketchup, mustard, salad dressings, nuts, BBQ sauce, breaded or processed meats, gourmet coffee and sausages can all present a problem. These foods are renowned for hidden carbs and you have got to check the label to make sure what you are getting on this diet.

Likewise, watch out in restaurants. They will sometimes use a watery sugar on the vegetables that will wreak havoc. Our society has got a sweet tooth and you are going to run into it at every turn during the weekdays. You will have to be especially careful during this Start-Up Phase as you get used to the diet and learn where the trouble spots may be.

Do Not Mix Diets

Again, the temptation may be big to mix diets combining the Metabolic Diet with aspects of other diets including the high carb and low fat diets, and putting them together in your own personal Frankenstein stew. Do not.

Many people will go on the Metabolic Diet but try to be true to their old high carb master. They will eat meat but it's all fish, chicken and turkey. While these foods may be quite nutritious and beneficial, even when used in the Metabolic Diet, they cannot be used as a total replacement for good, old-fashioned red meat. They just do not have enough fat.

What you end up doing by taking on the turkey/chicken/fish holy trinity is going on a high protein, low carb, low FAT diet. Along with being even harder to stay on than the Metabolic Diet, this diet will not get you the advantages you are looking for from the Metabolic Diet. You will not burn the fat like you should. You will not have the energy. You will not build the mass.

You need some red meat, and the more the better. You need the fat it provides. And you need to supplement your diet with other fats, such as the healthy omega-3 fatty acids including flax and fish oil. Do not shortchange yourself by trying to avoid fat (and certainly do not cut out healthy amounts of the essential fatty acids – like many do when on low fat diets) in some misled effort to stay true to forces in society who have labeled meat some kind of monster. This is simply not true.

Training in Start Up Phase

Start Up training should consist of some progressive circuit type training using a very light load for the first few sessions. Gradually increase the weight and resistance but not to the point where you are ever going all out. Repetitions should be in the 12 to 15 range all throughout this phase and the training time around one hour.

For example you could pick a combination of ten or more circuit and machine exercises and do one set of each and then do another set with some added weight or resistance.

Exercise	Reps	Sets
Leg Extensions	12-15	2
Leg Curl	12-15	2
Inner Thigh	12-15	2
Outer Thigh	12-15	2
Calf Raise	12-15	2
Abdominal	12-15	2
Butt Blaster Or Leg Press	12-15	2
Shoulder Press	12-15	2
Vertical Butterfly	12-15	2
Seated Chest	12-15	2
Bicep Curl	12-15	2
Lower Back	12-15	2
Seated Row	12-15	2
Triceps Push Down	12-15	2

Keys To Dieting Success In The Start Up Phase

1. Find the "maintenance" level were calories maintain your body weight (18 X Your Present Body Weight A Good Starting Point)
2. Take a fiber supplement
3. Watch for hidden carbs
4. Do not mix diets
5. The first week is the toughest – Stick It Out
6. Usually lasts 3-4 weeks

The First Week Is The Toughest

In the first week of the diet you will be going through the "metabolic shift" from being a carb and muscle-burning machine to being a fat burner and it can be difficult. While some people will suffer few symptoms, others will be very affected. The bowel irregularities we discussed above will come into play. You will also experience some fatigue and get foul or fruity smelling breath caused by an increase in the production of ketones, compounds that result from the initial steps of fat oxidation.

Emotionally, you could feel irritable and mentally foggy in the first week. You may suffer some very mild disorientation.

You can also experience pre-flu like symptoms where you feel like "something's coming on" or you are "fighting something off". Energy can drop and you can feel frequently hungry. Do not be alarmed. Basically, your body is just going through a readjustment phase. It will soon pass.

Unfortunately, many people will experience these difficulties and give up on the diet or increase their carbs too soon. They try it for a couple days and do not feel good and conclude "it doesn't work for me". They never break through the barrier to experience the "metabolic shift" and the increased energy and sense of well being it can bring.

That is why we urge you to STICK WITH IT DURING THE FIRST WEEK. Once you get through that first week, it's all downhill. You will start to feel better and better and the diet will be easier and easier. You will get to the point where you will feel so good the Metabolic Diet will seem like a revelation. You will not suffer those insulin ups and downs anymore. Energy will return. You will feel strong and lean and, in most cases, you will not be tempted to go back to the old, inferior way of eating. BUT YOU have GOT TO GET THROUGH THAT FIRST WEEK AND PAY SOME DUES TO EXPERIENCE THE BENEFITS.

Generally you will continue with the Start-Up Phase of the diet until you have got all your energy back and have no other symptoms. This will usually take 3-4 weeks and you will know when it's time. You will be feeling very, very good.

At this point you can move on to the next phase, the "mass phase" of the diet. But if you find you have got enough mass, you can stay at this phase for a while and then move on to a "cutting" phase as needed. The "start up" phase, without all the introductory facets, can be returned to when needed as a transition between the "mass" and "cutting" phases of the diet. As such, it can also properly be called the "maintenance" phase of the Metabolic Diet.

If you have problems getting things going and experience fatigue then make the necessary changes by going through the troubleshooting chart and guide on pages 81-83 in the Metabolic Diet book. Once you have straightened things out you can continue with the Mass Phase or if you are massive enough, you can go right to the cutting phase and begin to zero in on that weight loss and body shaping you have been dreaming of.

Supplements for the Start Up Phase

As I mentioned above, in the Start-Up Phase you should concentrate on making the metabolic shift and keeping everything else basically the same. As such, besides fiber supplements I usually do not suggest much else, other than a daily vitamin/mineral tablet, in this phase. If you are used to taking certain supplements on a regular basis you may want to continue doing so. Again, this phase is to get you into the Metabolic Diet and make that all-important shift from using carbs to using fats as your primary fuel. For this reason it's best to concentrate on making this shift and keeping other changes to a minimum.

Using my line of supplements as examples, supplements you could use include **MVM**, **Antiox** and **EFA+**. Also useful, and in some cases a must, as mentioned above is Regulate.

Regulate is an potent blend of natural soluble and insoluble fibers, plus probiotic ingredients, formulated for both preventing and treating constipation, frequent bowel movements, and other problems.

The various soluble fibers and other compounds contained in Regulate have also been found useful to:

- Maintain cholesterol levels that are already within normal range.
- Support a healthy heart.
- Increase natural insulin sensitivity.
- Has probiotic effects – promotes growth of beneficial bacteria in bowels.

As well, Regulate, by delaying gastric emptying and reducing the time to perceived fullness, is effective as an appetite suppressant. Taken before meals or whenever hungry, Regulate lessens your hunger and curbs cravings.

If you are feeling tired and generally having a hard time adjusting to the low carbs, and before you adjust your carb levels, try using Metabolic and Creatine Advantage to help get you through the rough spots.

Metabolic optimizes the effects of thyroid hormone, decreases cortisone levels, naturally increases levels of growth hormone and testosterone (in both men and women), and increases the body's natural insulin sensitivity. These effects increase weight and fat loss while maintaining or even increasing muscle mass.
Creatine Advantage keeps the energy system in high gear. Added amino acids and dipeptides allow a natural increase in the absorption and utilization of creatine and increase the volumizing, anticatabolic and anabolic effect of the formula. The added energy ingredients make Creatine Advantage the most advanced creatine and energy mix, one that will maximize energy, muscle mass and performance.

Mass Phase

This is the bread and butter phase of training. It's where you get to put on the muscle mass and start getting strong. You will not worry if you put on some fat in this stage because it's the muscle mass you are after. You will lose the fat later on and keep most of the muscle you have put on in this phase. Bottom line is that if you do not put on a load of muscle in this phase, you will not have any muscle to keep when you start dropping that bodyfat.

The idea behind this phase is to use a more structured approach to your training, and to increase the weight while decreasing the reps. The number of reps you do will vary but should be in the six to fifteen rep range, depending on the exercise and the bodypart being worked.

In this phase the exercises should concentrate on the big muscle masses. As such, it's the compound movements that you will be using, including squats, bench presses, rowing, and deadlifts. On the other hand you will also be working the smaller muscles especially the arm, forearm, neck and calves. You want to progressively move more weight but still keep the reps relatively high (at least relative to the Strength Phase).

The objective is to fatigue the muscles completely in every set but not to overload the musculature as far as the weight used. In this phase the training sets up the conditions for maximizing mass, while the diet meets the energy and macronutrient needs. In order to exhaust the muscles, especially as the weeks go by, you may have to use some special techniques, including cheat reps, partner assisted reps, partial reps, supersets, eccentric training and slow training, to keep the adaptation process in high gear.

The most important thing to remember during the mass phase is to keep the muscles working full out so you can maximize the increase in mass that results from your body adapting to the workload you put on it.

MASS PHASE

- Bulking up phase
- Not necessary if muscle mass is adequate and losing bodyfat more important.
- Hallmark of this phase is increasing muscle mass with some inevitable increase in bodyfat, although this increase should be kept to a minimum depending on your goals.

Training in the Mass Phase

It's best to concentrate on the big muscle masses as this results in the most overall muscle mass increase. This is done by using heavy-duty compound movements such as squats, bench presses, rowing, and deadlifts. That doesn't mean you cannot also do some more specialized exercises, ones that work the smaller muscles especially the arm, forearm, neck and calves. These, however, should be done after working the large muscle groups.

Although you should progressively increase the weight you use in each exercise, you should keep the reps in the 10 to 15 range. The workout time should be between one and one a half hours per training session.

Although initially you might be able to get away with training the whole body three times a week, later on as the workouts get more intense, you will likely split up the bodyparts and train each one twice a week or perhaps even once a week depending on the routine you use.

For example here's a 4 day split power and mass routine.

Tuesday	Wednesday
Legs: ➲ Squats ➲ Smith machine ➲ Leg presses ➲ Quad extensions ➲ Calf raises	**Chest and Delts:** ➲ Bench Presses ➲ Dumbbell bench presses ➲ Seated presses, bench presses and pec dec on circuit machines ➲ Lateral raises
Thursday	**Friday**
Back: ➲ Deadlifts ➲ Lat pulldowns ➲ Rowing ➲ Rowing on circuit machine ➲ Laybacks on circuit machine	**Arms:** ➲ Barbell curls ➲ Dumbbell curls ➲ Dips ➲ Triceps pressdown ➲ Forearm front and back bench curls ➲ Curls on circuit machine

Here's a 5 Day split routine with one bodypart worked per day. I have arbitrarily used Tuesday to Saturday as the workout days with Sunday and Monday off.

Tuesday	Wednesday
Back: ➲ Pull-up (chins) (3 sets max) ➲ Medium Grip Pulldown (3 X 12) ➲ Reverse Hyperextensions (3 X 12) ➲ Regular Deadlift (3 X 12) **Neck:** ➲ Shrugs (3 X12)	**Biceps:** ➲ Barbell Curl (3 X 12) ➲ Dumbbell Curl (3 X 12) ➲ Preacher Curl (3 X 12) **Triceps:** ➲ French Press (decline) (3 X 12) ➲ Triceps Dips (3 X max) ➲ Dumbbell Extension (3 X 12) ➲ Cable Pushdown (3 X 12) ➲ Close Grip Bench Press (3 X 12)
Thursday	**Friday**
Chest: ➲ Bench Press (3 X 12) ➲ Incline Bench Press (3 X 12) ➲ Incline Dumbbell Fly (3 X 12) ➲ Decline Bench Press (3 X 12) ➲ Cable Crossovers (3 X 12) ➲ Dumbbell Pullovers (2 X 12) ➲ Pec Deck (3 X 15)	**Thighs:** ➲ Squat (3 X 12) ➲ Leg Press (3 X 12) ➲ Lunge (3 X 12) ➲ Quad Extension (3 X 12) **Hams:** ➲ Hamstring Curl (3 X 12) **Calves:** ➲ Standing Calf Raise (4 X 12) ➲ Seated Calf Raise (4 X 12)
Saturday	
Shoulders: ➲ Military Press – front/back each ➲ (2 X 12) ➲ Side Raise (2 X 12) ➲ Bent-over Side Raise (3 X 12) ➲ Front Raises (3 X 12)	

Nutrition for the Mass Phase

This phase is similar to the "bulking up" phase most bodybuilders are familiar with. As usual, you will be increasing your calorie intake. On the Metabolic Diet, your goal should be to ALLOW YOUR BODY WEIGHT TO INCREASE TO 15 PERCENT ABOVE YOUR IDEAL WEIGHT.

When we use the term "ideal weight" we are talking about what you consider to be your optimum ripped or even contest weight and you have got to be practical about it. For example, if you are a competitive bodybuilder and you have been competing at 200 pounds for 4-5 years and then say your ideal weight is 315, that is not practical. More reasonable would be to take that ideal weight up to 215 or so and increase your weight to 15 percent above this, or 250 pounds, in this phase.

Realize that if you go hog wild, eat like crazy and end up going 30 percent above your "ideal weight" your body will end up being 15 percent bodyfat or more. That is not what we are looking for here. The Metabolic Diet is designed to get you more muscle and limit bodyfat. Even though you will experience an increase in lean mass and put on less fat than you would on another diet, you have still got to exercise some discipline.

As far as the specifics of the diet itself, they are the same on this phase as on the others. You will be sticking to the weekday high protein, higher fat, weekend carb load plan. The only change will be in the amount of calories you eat. If you want to get to a level 15 percent above your ideal weight, you are obviously going to have to eat more.

To achieve this, the bodybuilder should consume 25 CALORIES PER POUND and 55 CALORIES PER KG OF BODYWEIGHT DESIRED EVERY DAY. In the example above, the bodybuilder wants to get to 250 pounds so he will be eating 6,250 calories (25 X 250) a day. When you consider that he's probably been on a 3,600 calorie diet before that, you can see the tremendous increase in calories he's going to experience.

This can present a big problem for athletes who have trouble gaining weight. They are not used to eating and do not really have big appetites. They may think they are eating huge amounts but they are not. They will find themselves at 6,000 calories one day and down at 1,500 a few days later. You ask them what happened and all they will say is "I wasn't hungry."

You cannot do that on this diet. You have got to be consistent. If you want, you can multiply that 6,250 calories times 7 and make your goal 43,750 for the week. That way you can vary some from day to day, for example eat 7,500 calories one day and 5,000 the next, but by the end of the week you have got to be at the 43,750 calorie level. Keep a diary or some other record of calories eaten and make sure that you are doing it.

Usually most bodybuilders find that they can take in more calories on the weekend than they can on weekdays. That is OK as long as you stay within your weekly total calories. For example if your goal is your goal is 43,750 for the week, you might want to average out at 5,000 calories or so a day on weekdays and up it to 9,000 to 10,000 calories or so on Saturday and Sunday.

KEYS TO SUCCESS IN THE MASS PHASE

1. Increase bodyweight to 15 percent above your "ideal" contest weight.
2. Eat 25 calories per pound of "ideal" weight daily.
3. If you have trouble eating enough, make calories a weekly, rather than daily, goal.
4. Bodyfat shouldn't rise above the 10 percent level.
5. End the "Mass Phase" when you reach your "ideal" weight or rise to the 10 percent bodyfat level, whichever comes first.
6. Whether you have reached your "ideal" weight or not, the "Mass Phase" must cease at least 12 weeks before a contest.
7. A gain of 2 pounds per week is best.

Controlling Bodyfat

Of course, bodyfat is also of critical importance here. Some athletes will gain more bodyfat than others at similar calorie levels. As well, depending on personal goals, some individuals will not mind gaining a little more fat if it means more muscle and strength. While the 10% rule is best for competitive bodybuilders, and actually any athlete who competes in a specific weight class, other athletes may be willing to go higher and find that even up to 15% is acceptable, especially if it means more hypertrophy and strength. Just keep in mind that if you let your bodyfat levels get too high, it will be that much harder to get it off.

Since most athletes want to maximize muscle mass and strength, and minimize bodyfat, we will use the competitive bodybuilding model to discuss reaching their weight and muscle mass gains during the Mass Phase.

We have found that most bodybuilders can maintain a 10 percent bodyfat level relatively easily if properly utilizing the Metabolic Diet. This is also a good level to stay at to keep fat in check in any preparation for competitive bodybuilding. That is why we advise those on the Metabolic Diet to keep close track of their bodyfat level and do not let it go above this 10 percent level.

With this in mind the goal in the "Mass Phase" is to continue eating and gaining weight until you either reach a level 15 percent above your "ideal weight" or hit 10 percent bodyfat, whichever comes first. Chances are, no matter what comes first, you will get the mass you want on this anabolically supercharged diet. It's not like the old days with the high carb diet where you have got to gain so much weight and fat to get mass.

You have to use your head here, though. If you find yourself still gaining weight but haven't reached your "ideal" and your contest is 12 weeks away it's time to stop the "Mass Phase". It's time to begin cutting to properly prepare yourself for the contest regardless of weight. In this way, time before a contest joins bodyfat and weight as a determinant in how long you will stay in this phase.

On the other hand, I know many bodybuilders who have come to believe they should gain mass quickly but I do not agree with this. 2 pounds a week is good enough. If you can gain 2, you will not gain a lot of fat during the week on the Metabolic Diet. It will be mostly muscle. Though I'd vary this one pound plus or minus given individual differences, I think 2 pounds a week is the best benchmark for bulking up.

Mass Phase Duration Can Vary

Not that the Mass Phase cannot be hurried, but for the competitive bodybuilder, you always want to maintain right about 10 percent bodyfat. That way you can get in contest shape fast. I have seen people go through a 20-week cycle in which they have bulked up for 8 weeks (3 pounds a week), skip the other phases and then use 12 weeks for cutting (1-2 pounds a week). Though they bulked for only 8 weeks and cut for 12, their weight was still above what it was for the contest before. And they were as cut if not more so.

The whole goal here is to come into a contest a little better than before you were on the diet. This may mean only 3-4 pounds. Or, in more long-term training, it could be 25. The big thing is, EVERYBODY MAKES PROGRESS WITH THIS DIET. To those people who have been the same for 15 years I say, here's a way to break out.

Some bodybuilders prefer to point for a big contest, like a Mr. Olympia, and take the whole year to do it. That can easily be done on this diet, too. You may want to mass for 20 weeks, maintain and consolidate your muscle gains by going into the Strength Phase for 10 weeks, and cut for 20 weeks, gaining 60 pounds and losing 40 over the course of a year. You will come in 20 pounds ahead of where you were last year and be looking great.

For those who aren't after the really low bodyfat levels that competitive bodybuilders have to reach you might want to end your mass phase when you reach your ideal weight or rise to the percent bodyfat level you feel comfortable with (usually anywhere from 10 to 15 percent).

Weekly Weight Gains

You may see big fluctuations in weight, especially at the beginning of the diet, as a result of your weekly carb loads. All the extra carbs and water can make for a gain of from 5-10 pounds between Friday and Monday.

If this happens, do not stress out. It's natural. When you go back on the Metabolic Diet on Monday you will immediately begin shedding those pounds, which are mostly water. Monday-Wednesday you will be cleaning out much of what you put into your body on the weekend. By Wednesday you should be pretty well flushed out and feeling good again. Depending on what phase of the diet you are on, you can manipulate calories so you get either the weekly weight gain or loss you are looking for by Friday.

If you are after maximum mass, without putting on too much bodyfat, you can do this by dramatically increasing your calories on the weekend and keeping the increases moderate during the weekdays. For example a friend of mine who went to well over 300 pounds while in the mass phase ate over 12,000 calories a day on both Saturday and Sunday. He kept this up until he was at the bodyweight he wanted and then dealt with the increased fat by going on the Cutting Phase for a longer period of time. He felt that doing it this way allowed him to hit the competition with more muscle and just as ripped than if he didn't gain the extra weight during the Mass Phase.

EXTREME VARIANCE

- Extreme Mass Phase.
- Huge intake of carbs and calories over the weekend. Up to 12,000 calories on both Saturday and Sunday.

Supplements for the Mass Phase

In the Mass Phase it's the food that counts more than the supplements. Getting your quota of low carb calories will supply you with much of what you need to pack on size and muscle. However, several of the more general supplements, including one or more of **MVM** (my complete vitamin/mineral/nutrient supplement), **Antiox** (my antioxidant mix), and **EFA+** (my essential fatty acid formula that contains much more than just the essential fatty acids), should be used on a regular basis, and others, such as **ReNew**, Regulate, Joint Support, LoCarb MRP and Sports bars should be used as needed. For example if you are running into training problems, joint pain, injuries, and overtraining, I recommend that you use **Joint Support** and/or ReNew. Also the **LoCarb MRP** and **Sports Bars** can be extremely useful for snacks or after meals to help you reach your calorie goals in a healthy, low carb way.

Also, if you reach a plateau in this phase, especially in your training, or if you want to gain mass faster, you might want to use **Exersol** to maximize your training efforts. Exersol is a three-phase exercise-oriented nutritional support system that takes the guesswork out of what supplements to use before, during and after training. As the most scientifically advanced and sophisticated exercise orientated nutritional support system ever formulated, its use is invaluable for anyone who wants to lose bodyfat and build muscle. For more details see Appendix One.

In fact, for more information on all the supplements mentioned in this book, see Appendix One. Also check them out regularly on **www.MetabolicDiet.com**. There you will find the most up to date information on my evolving Signature Series line of nutritional supplements that I formulated especially for the Anabolic Solution and the Anabolic/Metabolic Diet. These supplements are unique and effective and cover the complete gamut of supplement needs. For example Power Drink fills a gap that is been overlooked by all the other supplement companies. While they are absorbed in what to use before and after training, and rightly so, they are missing one of the most important opportunities for maximizing the results you get from training.

A Quick Guide To Supplements To Use In And Around Training.

Resolve or Resolve Competition, Power Drink and **Amino** take care of the pretraining, during training, and immediate post training periods (see **Exersol** in the Appendix). However, to round off training supplementation we should also add **MRP LoCarb**. This meal substitute, taken within an hour or so after training, will maximize muscle mass and recovery for anyone following the Metabolic Diet, better than any other post workout product. If you are in the Mass Phase then you can mix it with milk (taking the carb content into account) and if you are in the cutting phase then taking it with water works best.

The combination of specific proteins, fats and minimal carbs in MRP LoCarb is engineered to dramatically increase protein synthesis, maximize muscle intracellular triglycerides and glycogen, while at the same time limiting fat formation and storage, and increase recovery. The special blend of proteins in MRP LoCarb, similar to the one that is in the Myosin Protein blend, maximizes protein synthesis and minimize protein breakdown for several hours.

Also, while taking in fat post workout will slow protein absorption in those that are carb adapted, it doesn't in people who are fat adapted, such as those on the Metabolic Diet. In fact taking in some fat is beneficial as not only doesn't it slow down protein absorption and thus allows maximum protein synthesis, but it also increases intracellular fatty acid content, resulting in increased muscle size and increased endurance and recovery.

SUPPLEMENTS IN AND AROUND TRAINING

Prior to Training
- Resolve or Resolve Competition

During Training
- Power Drink

Right After Training
- Amino

Within an hour of Training
- MRP LoCarb in Water, or with Milk

Power Drink – Filling the Gap

We all know that during training muscle is broken down. Most people believe that this breakdown is a necessary part of training. After all you have to break muscle tissue down before you can build it up. Do not you? Unfortunately that is one of the most stubborn training myths. Muscle breakdown isn't what provides the adaptation stimulus for increasing muscle size. It's the damage done to the muscle cell structure and the subsequent adaptation to that damage that determines the muscle building response. You do not have to break down the muscle at all to get this response in full force. In fact doing so is counter productive. The more muscle you keep from breaking down, and the more you increase protein synthesis, the better the results from your training. Taking Power Drink while you are training will put you miles ahead of everyone else who just uses water or at best a carbohydrate low protein drink.

As well, Power Drink, because of its positive effects on the fat burning hormones and mechanisms actually allows you to burn more bodyfat while you are training. And with the other ingredients in Power Drink you can train harder and longer and know that you have a powerful ally that will help you make good use of all that hard work.
Bottom line is that Power Drink is a revolutionary new concept in training drinks. This drink provides the nutrients necessary to increase muscle size and decrease bodyfat. By providing all the necessary ingredients to feed working muscles and shift the use of bodyfat as the energy source for training, Power Drink dramatically increases the positive effects of training, allows you train longer and harder, and increases recovery.
Power Drink is ideal for both those who want to increase muscle size and lose bodyfat and those who simply want to lose weight and bodyfat but maintain the muscle they now have.
Besides the hefty dose (44 grams) of the best quality proteins available anywhere, Power Drink also contains amino acids, electrolytes and other ingredients that will replace and replenish nutrients and fluid lost through exercise, prevent muscle cramps, and increase training time and efficiency.

Dr. D's Metabolic Shake

I often recommend combinations of various supplements for the different training phases. One example is a metabolic shake that some people find very useful as sort of a super shake for all the phases.

To make Dr. D's Metabolic Shake, take one packet of APT MRP LoCarb Shake, one to two scoops of each of the APT Myosin Protein and APT Creatine Advantage and blend to taste. This super shake gives you a 1-2-3 punch for maximum effect on muscle mass, strength and fat loss. The two versions of this shake are described below:

1. **Dr. D's Metabolic Shake**: Uses only the three mixed together to minimize carb intake and especially suited for the Cutting Phase.
   - APT MRP LoCarb
   - APT Creatine Advantage
   - ATP Myosin Protein
2. **Dr. D's Carb-Enhanced Metabolic Shake**: Includes extra carbs and is especially suited for the Mass and Strength Phases:
   - APT MRP LoCarb
   - APT Creatine Advantage
   - ATP Myosin Protein
   - Add fruit and/or scoop of ice cream to desired carb level

Nighttime Protein Supplements

Grow muscle while you sleep. Is that possible or just hype? In fact it is and it's due to the dynamics of sleep and exercise.

The fact is that you do not build muscles while you are exercising but while you are resting. Following a single bout of resistance training in healthy males, Chesley and colleagues found that muscle protein synthesis in the biceps brachii remained elevated for up to 24 hours postexercise.[95] During this recovery period the inhibition of protein synthesis in previously less active muscles and fibers makes it possible to concentrate the adaptive protein synthesis for structures that performed the highest load. That means that the muscle you worked the most get the most attention and grow more in order to adapt to that day's exercise.

If all this is the case then why do we all neglect that part of our 24 hour day when we rest the most? That is right, I am talking about that forgotten seven or eight hours while you sleep. Why do we fast during the night and then try to make it up with a meal to break that fast? Having a good break-fast just will not cut it. We need to think about all those wasted hours between the time we go to bed to the time we get up and break our usual fast.

During our night time fast, since it cannot get the energy and nutrients it needs from food, your body gets them any way it can, usually be sacrificing some of your muscle for the amino acids your body needs for it's various functions and for fuel.

The other side of all this is that if you are short on the building blocks that make up muscle, then you are not going to build muscle as well as losing it. That is a double whammy that will knock your muscle mass down.

We already know that the body's primed for growth and repair while we are sleeping. So what we need to do is to give the body the chance and the material to do its job. If you do it right, you can make maximum use of that beauty sleep to grow muscle, repair and rejuvenate the body and mind, and lose bodyfat.

Anabolic and Catabolic Influences for Increasing Muscle Mass

It's important to understand what's involved in increasing muscle mass. There is a delicate balance between protein synthesis (building muscle) and protein catabolism (breaking down muscle). Both processes go on simultaneously and it's the balance between the two that decides whether or not you are going to gain or lose muscle mass.

It's also important to understand that even if protein synthesis increases all during sleep because of an increase in anabolic hormones, the natural tendency of the body is to break down muscle in the postabsorptive phase – when there is no longer any food in the GI tract that is being absorbed. The body needs a constant supply of energy and nutrients and if this supply is not forthcoming from dietary intake then it takes what it needs from body stores and the breakdown of tissue, especially muscle.

It's the net gain in protein accretion that is important, not the degree of either protein synthesis or degradation. Even in states in which extensive protein degradation, as long as protein synthesis is greater, then we are in positive protein balance and building muscle. So it makes just as much sense to try and decrease protein degradation as to increase protein synthesis, and makes the most sense if you can do both at the same time.

Processes that decrease catabolism are called anticatabolic in that they decrease or even prevent muscle catabolism. It's important to realize that muscle mass can decrease as a result of decreased catabolism, either physiologically or through the use of anticatabolic agents, just as much as from anabolism. In fact if catabolism is not checked it can easily outstrip any anabolic processes and result in muscle loss.

The Missing Link

So if you eat right, train hard, and take your supplements and you are still not growing, you better start taking your sleep time more seriously because that is just may be the anabolic primer you are missing.

Most of us take sleeping for granted. We go to bed and wake up in the morning with little care of what goes on in between. But if you are a bodybuilder and you want to maximize the effects of your training you should care because what you do, or more specifically what you are not doing, while you sleep may be sabotaging all your hard training.

The first thing you have to do is to make sure you are getting your fair share of sleep. Look at sleep as a "do not disturb" sign for out bodies and mind and make sure you are not short changing yourself by not getting enough of it. Without enough sleep both our bodies and minds, and our metabolism are adversely affected.

We live in a society that is in a frenzy 24/7, and few people value a good nights sleep. That is because we have so many demands on us that we are always looking for a few extra hours to catch up. And most of us cut back on our sleep to gain that time. As such, sleep deprivation is all too common in our culture, with disastrous consequences on our mental and physical health. And as important, at least for us, on our ability to gain muscle and lose bodyfat.

Besides all the rejuvenating effects of sleep on our brain and nervous system, many of the body's cells also show increased production and reduced breakdown of proteins during sleep. Since proteins are the building blocks needed for cell growth and for repair of damage from factors like training, stress and even ultraviolet rays, the time we sleep should be optimized to get the best results.

Phases of Sleep

Although we do not pay much attention to sleep, we all know that there are times when we sleep deeply and times when we sleep lightly and have dreams. Actually there are five stages of sleep that are repeated in a cycle several times during the night. For our purposes, however, we can simplify them into two stages, deep sleep and light or rapid eye movement (REM) sleep.

When we are first falling asleep, we drift in and out of sleep and can be awakened easily. This progresses into the first deep sleep of the night, and the time in which there are changes in the regulatory influences and growth hormone peaks.[96,97] In deep sleep we are almost in a coma, eye movements and muscle activity stop altogether and brain waives become slower until in the deepest sleep, the brain is producing delta waves exclusively. It appears that it's in this mode that your body goes into a repair and rebuild or "rejuvenation" mode.

When you progress from deep sleep to REM sleep, you are actually beginning to wake up. In REM, breathing becomes more rapid, irregular and shallow, eyes jerk rapidly in various directions, muscles that are already limp from deep sleep become temporarily paralyzed (likely to prevent us from acting out our dreams), heart rate increases and blood pressure rises. REM is the sleep from which dreams are born and persons awakened during REM will usually be able to remember some details of their dreams.

In REM sleep neuronal messages from the motor cortex of the brain are blocked at the brain stem. As a result, your muscles are completely relaxed and you are unable to move. Thus, REM sleep is characterized by an active brain, dreaming away, in what amounts to a "paralyzed" body.

While there is been a lot of research on what goes on when we sleep, there are a lot of gaps in our knowledge. On top of that many of the studies reveal contradictory or inconclusive findings. So for the purposes of this article, while I will be drawing on solid scientific research, I will also be extrapolating from known facts, and mixing this in with my own feelings and opinions.

So What Can You Do?

For years I have felt that we were missing the boat when it came to maximizing muscle mass because we ignored overcoming the nightly decrease in muscle growth caused by post-absorptive muscle catabolism. Well no more. We have the technology to provide full spectrum night time nutrition that will fill this crucial gap.

So what's to do? Well there are lots of factors to consider. Ideally what you want to accomplish is to make sleep time growth time by using a six-pronged approach.

Factors to Consider

1. Getting a good night's sleep.
2. Increasing the use of fatty acids and decrease the use of muscle protein (and thus decrease muscle breakdown) for gluconeogenesis and oxidation as fuel.
3. Manipulating the anabolic and catabolic hormones to maximize protein synthesis and minimize protein breakdown during sleep.
4. Increasing cell hydration (volumizing) and as such stimulating protein synthesis.

5. Enhancing Immune System to decrease catabolic cytokines and other factors.

6. Minimizing the postabsorptive phase by modulating nutrient absorption and effects.

First of all you want to make sure that you get a good nights sleep, with solid and refreshing deep sleep phases and REM sleep phases. The deep sleep is important to create that night-time GH peak, and the REM for it's cognitive and immune system rejuvenation. In fact sleep deprivation, something all of us go through with the hectic pace we keep, can not only deprive you of the benefits you should be getting from exercise, but it can impact all areas of your life including your ability to work, your body's ability to defend itself and your maintenance of a positive attitude.

Exercise can affect sleep quality. Although there are a number of inconsistencies in the literature,[98] it seems that while light exercise favors sleep and enhances all the sleep phases,[99] more intense exercise can have adverse effects on both sleep latency (the time it takes to fall asleep) and sleep quality.[100101]

So sometimes it's hard to get to sleep and get a good night's sleep after a hard workout. A combination of just the right ingredients taken before bed will ensure that you get a good shot at a restful and rejuvenation night's sleep.

Optimizing the Hormones

Secondly you want to optimize the anabolic and minimize the catabolic influences, as well as maximizing fat burning. That can be done by manipulating and maximizing the sex hormones, especially testosterone, and both GH and IGF-1, at the same time as insulin. As well, you should lower cortisol.

HORMONE MANIPULATION

- Testosterone – increase
- Cortisol – decrease
- Growth Hormone – increase
- IGF-I – increase
- Insulin – increase amount and sensitivity
- Thyroid – control

Under normal conditions, testosterone, GH and subsequently IGF-I all increase during sleep. Keep in mind that high levels of all three, equals positive nitrogen balance and muscle growth.

The night time increase in all three hormones, including the GH peak during slow wave sleep,[102] has been well established.[103] In fact in part because of these increases, sleep may be the prime period for anabolic activity.

However, it has also been shown that heavy resistance training[104] and long duration exercise[105] may adversely affect testosterone levels, and night time GH, IGF-I and cortisol release . As such it's important to augment GH release in the crucial 24 hours after training, especially at night.

Augmenting the night time anabolic hormones is even more important as we age. Not only do the general level of these hormones decline significantly and steadily after the third decade, but the quality of sleep and the night time surge of GH and IGF-I are adversely affected by aging.[106,107] So it's also important to make sure we are sleeping well and to naturally augment these hormones as we age.

Anabolic Effects of Increasing Cellular Hydration

Using certain compounds to increase cell hydration and cell volume is also a good strategy. That is because cell volume homeostasis involves the integration of events that allow cell hydration to play a physiologic role as a regulator of cell function, including protein synthesis.[108]

Taurine, glutamine and the electrolytes sodium and potassium are transported into cells with a resulting osmotic swelling of the cell that produces an increase in cell volume. It is generally felt that the mechanism through which there is an activation of key enzymes in these metabolic pathways involves the compound-induced cell swelling and results in an increase in protein synthesis.[109]

Enhancing the Immune System

While a good nights sleep enhances the immune system and decreases the production of inflammatory cytokines,[110] the use of certain compounds can increase this response. Enhancing the immune system decreases catabolic influences and improved net protein balance. Several compounds can enhance the immune system and include glutamine, glutathione, vitamins A and E, whey, casein and milk isolates protein, and colostrum.

For example, glutamine acts as a primary fuel for certain immune cells, which are activated under stress conditions. High intensity exercise, while considered a beneficial form of stress, still exerts a glutamine-depleting effect on muscle. Exogenous glutamine enhances the immune system to decrease catabolic cytokines and result in a positive nitrogen balance and increased recovery. Colostrum on the other hand contains several immune components and also contains IGF-I, an anabolic growth factor.

The Dreaded Postabsorptive Phase

Next you want to minimize the postabsorptive phase by making what you take before bed last as long as possible. Ideally for the full time you are sleeping.

The human body, through metabolic and hormonal controls, has evolved to meet the continuous metabolic needs of the body even though eating and thus provision of essential nutrients is intermittent.

During and after feeding while food is still being absorbed, in the postabsorptive period (after a meal has been almost completely digested and the resulting nutrients absorbed into the body – usually 3 to 4 hours after a meal – the transition from the postprandial to the fasting state occurs within 6-12 hours after a meal) and even under fasting conditions (as long as the fasting state is not extensive), the body tends to keep a constant energy output by utilizing dietary sources when available and at other times by mobilizing internal substrates (glycogen, cellular and bodyfat, cellular protein) that can be used as energy sources.

Postabsorptive energy sources include circulating glucose, fatty acids, and triglycerides, liver and muscle glycogen, the branched chain amino acids (used by skeletal muscle) and the amino acids alanine and glutamine (released from skeletal muscle and used for gluconeogenesis, in the case of glutamine directly as fuel by the immune system and gastrointestinal tract).[111,112] In a normal 70-kg man these postabsorptive energy sources provide up to 1200 kcal (800 calories from carbohydrate sources). These sources can be exhausted in less than 12 hours if no other food is consumed.

In an individual that is dieting to lose weight or in an athlete that is limiting both caloric and fat intake in order to maximize lean body mass and minimize bodyfat, these sources may amount to less than 500 kcal since liver and muscle glycogen levels as well as circulating triglycerides and fatty acids are often limited.

In these cases the postabsorptive phase can be avoided by loading up on protein and amino acids before bed. This provides the body with both slow (for long term protein absorption and delays the postabsorptive phase) and fast proteins. The fast proteins allow for a protein peak early in the sleep process and act as an added stimulus for the GH peak, which in turn increases long term IGF-I secretion. There is also a decrease in the formation of glucose through gluconeogenesis, a process by which glucose is formed from other substrates, mainly lactate, pyruvate, glycerol and amino acids.[113,114,115] The end result is an increase in the use of fatty acids and ketones by the body, which in turn spares muscle from being broken down and increases the loss of bodyfat.

Ideally there should be no postabsorptive phase and all the anabolic and anti-catabolic effects of the various hormones should be maximized (through a synergistic action of testosterone, insulin, GH, IGF-I and thyroid), and the catabolic effects of cortisol minimized at a time when the availability of nutrients is maximal. Creating this ideal environment for muscle growth requires both knowledge and dedication.

We know that the availability of amino acids is both anabolic and anticatabolic per se, even when hormones are not optimized, and more so when they are. The lack of amino acids leads to a catabolic response as muscle tissue is broken down to supply the body with the nutrients and energy it needs during sleep.

So it is important to maintain positive "nitrogen balance" in the body while sleeping. When you do and conditions are right so that your rate of protein synthesis exceeds your rate of degradation, and you maintain a positive nitrogen balance, you can grow while you sleep.

So what we need to do is to try to have a continual supply of exogenous amino acids available through the night. This isn't possible with just using the foods and supplements now available. Also eating a big meal before bed, to try and stretch out how long food is absorbed, can be counter productive in that first of all it can make it uncomfortable to get to sleep, secondly it may decrease that important GH spike that usually occurs a few hours after you fall asleep, and perhaps more importantly, decrease night time levels of IGF-I.

You could always get up half way through the night and eat but doing so would be disruptive and likely lead to disturbed sleep and thus, for the reasons we have already mentioned, be counter productive.

What's needed is to create an anabolic, anticatabolic environment that will spare muscle by providing alternate fuel during sleep and as such allow the body to grow muscle and lose bodyfat during sleep.

Battling The Postabsorptive Phase With A Combination Of Proteins And Amino Acids

- Whey – fast protein – increase GH spike, Increase insulin.
- Casein – slow protein – delay postabsorptive phase.
- Peptides and amino acids including glutamine peptides, glutamine, and the branched chain amino acids, including leucine.

Summary

Converting your night-time down time to the plus side with just the right combination of supplements will do you and your body a world of good by:

- Decreasing muscle catabolism
- Increasing muscle anabolism
- Accelerating the breakdown and burning of bodyfat
- Increasing metabolic and muscular recovery
- Decreasing the effects of overtraining
- Increasing repair of over stressed and injured tissues
- Increasing sleep quality and restorative effects

NitAbol is a combination of three supplements that will maximize protein synthesis and increase fat oxidation while you sleep.

Strength Phase

This phase is an intermediate phase between the classical Mass or Bulk Phase and the Cutting or Definition Phase.

The goals of the Strength Phase are to maintain most of the weight and all of the muscle mass gained in the Mass Phase. During this phase we are after increases in strength to match the increased muscle mass. The raison d'être of the Strength Phase for bodybuilders is to consolidate muscle mass gains by increasing musculoskeletal strength. Increasing strength increases muscle protein retention and results in muscle that is denser. As a result, increasing strength to match increased muscle mass results in increased muscle mass retention in the Cutting Phase.

Training in the Strength Phase

In this phase we use a powerlifting type of approach to training concentrating again on the heavy-duty compound movements such as the squat, flat bench press, incline bench press, high pulls, deadlifts, bent over rowing, lat pulldowns, and chins, The main emphasis it to increase strength and use more weight with fewer repetitions than in the Mass Phase.

While the objective is still to fatigue the muscles completely in every set the emphasis is on doing this with heavier weights and fewer repetitions than in the Mass Phase. In the transition between the Mass and Strength Phases you simply begin to increase the weight and decrease the reps. The number of reps you do will vary but should be in the six to ten rep range, depending on the exercise and the bodypart being worked.

The objective is to fatigue the muscles completely by overloading the muscles as far as the weight used. In this phase the training sets up the conditions for consolidating muscle mass, while the diet meets the specific energy and macronutrient needs of this phase. As in the Mass Phase, in order to work the muscles adequately, especially as the weeks go by, you may have to use some special techniques, including mainly partner assisted reps (usually for only one or two reps maximum), or the use of chains and elastic bands, in order to keep the adaptation process in high gear.

Because you need more rest between sets, workout time in the Strength Phase is usually longer than in any of the other phases, usually a minimum of one and a half hours up to 2 hours. On the other hand, training frequency is less because it takes longer to recover from the workouts.

The most important thing to remember during the Strength Phase is consistently increase the weight used and to max out weight wise every workout. This keeps the muscles working to their strength capacity and consolidates the existing muscle mass.

An example of a 4 day split strength routine:

Tuesday	Wednesday
➲ Wide grip bench press ➔ 5 sets of 6 reps ➲ Narrow grip incline bench press – about 30 degrees ➔ 5 sets of 6 reps	➲ Rowing 4 sets of 6 reps ➲ Deadlift from below knees on Smith machine ➔ to maximum triple ➲ Seated rows ➔ 3 sets 8 reps
Friday	**Saturday**
➲ Barbell curls ➔ 6 sets of 8 reps ➲ Lying triceps presses ➔ 6 sets of 8 reps	➲ Regular bar squats ➔ 4 sets of 6 reps ➲ 1/2 squats on Smith machine ➔ 4 sets of 8 reps

Duration of the Strength Phase

The Strength Phase can last anywhere from a minimum of three weeks to a maximum of six weeks. Less than three weeks doesn't give the body enough time to solidify the muscle gains of the Mass Phase. And I have found that carrying on the Strength Phase beyond six weeks can, because of the intensity of the workouts, result in overtraining and injuries.

Nutrition for the Strength Phase

During this phase, an intermediate phase between the classical Mass or Bulk Phase and the Cutting or Definition Phase, we go through the process of increasing strength and solidifying the muscle mass gains of the Mass Phase. The nutrition goals in the Strength Phase is to maintain much of the weight and solidify all of the muscle mass gained during the Mass Phase, and ideally to increase muscle mass marginally, while at the same time maximizing the strength that would normally go along with the increased weight and muscle mass.

During this phase the bodybuilder should consume between 17 and 25 calories per day per pound or 37 and 55 calories per kg of the top bodyweight he or she attained during the Mass Phase. You start at the high level and from there cut back 1-2 calories per pound per week, or 2-4 calories per Kg per week until weight stabilizes. Then keep calories at that level. The amount of calories you cut depends on the Mass Phase weight you achieved. The higher your weight, the more calories you cut.

Using the same example, the 250 lb bodybuilder will now cut back roughly 2 calories per pound per week. That means that the first week of the Strength Phase he will take in 23 calories per pound of bodyweight or 23 * 250 = 5,750 calories per day. The following week he will take in 21 calories per pound of bodyweight or 5,250 calories per day. The third week 19 calories per pound of bodyweight or 4,750 calories per day. The fourth week 17 calories per pound of bodyweight or 4,250 calories per day and so on.

Once your weight stabilizes so that you are no longer gaining weight, keep the calories at that level or just slightly above or below until you go into the Cutting Phase.

DIETARY PROTEIN AND FAT

- **Dietary protein intake should be at the same level, or perhaps even higher, with a lower level of dietary fat intake as compared to the intakes in the Mass Phase.**
- Thus you as you cut calories it's fat calories and thus dietary fat intake that decreases.

Keys To Success In The Strength Phase

1. Stabilize your muscle mass gained through the Mass Phase.
2. Bodyfat shouldn't rise above the levels of the Mass Phase.
3. In the first week of the Strength Phase start cutting back from the 25 calories per pound of the Mass Phase. Cut back 2 cal per pound per week until your weight stabilizes.
4. Dietary protein intake should be at the same level with a lower level of dietary fat intake as compared to the intakes in the Mass Phase.
5. For maximum results, the use of nutritional supplements is a must.

Supplements for the Strength Phase

➲ Daily calories are decreasing and training intensity is increasing.

➲ The increased use of nutritional supplements makes up for any deficiencies, and increases the anabolic and fat burning effects of exercise.

In the Strength Phase, the supplements are more important than in the Start-Up and Mass Phases. It's still important to get your quota of low carb calories and dietary protein to supply you with much of what you need to solidify your increased muscle mass (by increasing muscle protein content and fiber density) and start getting ready to decrease your bodyfat. However, because the daily calories have decreased substantially over the Mass Phase, and your training intensity is increasing, supplementing your diet with some targeted supplements will allow you to make better progress.

As such you will need more than just your basic one a day vitamin and mineral tablet. **MVM** (my complete vitamin/mineral/nutrient supplement), **Antiox** (my antioxidant mix), and **EFA+** (my essential fatty acid formula that contains much more than just the essential fatty acids), should be used on a regular basis.

At this point **Exersol** (made up of Resolve, Power Drink and Amino) is a must. See the Appendix for details.

ReNew, **Regulate**, **Joint Support**, **LoCarb MRP** and **Sports Bars** can be used as needed.

For more information on these supplements see the supplement sections in the chapters describing the Mass and Cutting Phases, and the chapter Doing It Naturally. For complete information on these products log on to **www.MetabolicDiet.com**.

But besides the above supplements, the Strength Phase demands a more sophisticated array. At this time it's usually necessary to supplement the diet with additional "lean" protein and to make up the added protein calories by decreasing dietary fat. As well, we need to use three or four new formulations to maximize the anaerobic and aerobic energy systems and the anabolic drive.

- Myosin Protein allows you to keep protein levels up at a time when it might be difficult to take in enough protein from foods while at the same time cutting calories. It's an advanced synergistic blend of high quality protein powders including a specially developed source of glutamine peptides. Myosin Protein Complex, containing both fast and slowly absorbed proteins, is engineered to increase protein synthesis and decrease muscle breakdown by a direct effect, by increasing the anabolic and decreasing the catabolic hormones, and by providing the body with an increased immune response to combat overtraining and maximize the anabolic and fat burning effects of exercise. We use a variety of the highest quality protein powder to make use of the special characteristics of each and thus enhancing their overall effect while at the same time eliminating their relative disadvantages. Because of the gentle processes used to isolate the various proteins, the formula maintains the beneficial immune and other effects of the undenatured whey, casein and soy proteins.
- **Creatine Advantage** keeps the energy system in high gear despite the decreased caloric intake. As well, by increasing endogenous levels of phosphocreatine, Creatine Advantage increases the immediately available energy that is so necessary to fuel the Strength Phases' increased exercise intensity. Added amino acids and dipeptides allow a natural increase in the absorption and utilization of creatine and increase the volumizing, anticatabolic and anabolic effect of the formula. The added energy ingredients make Creatine Advantage the most advanced creatine and energy mix on the market today and one that will maximize muscle mass and performance.
- **TestoBoost** contains several natural ingredients and is designed to improve natural testosterone formation, and decrease any potential side effects from conversion of testosterone to estrogens and dihydrotestosterone. By boosting the body's natural testosterone, TestoBoost increases muscle mass, decreases bodyfat and increases sexual desire.
- **GHboost** is formulated to increase muscle mass and decrease bodyfat by enhancing the body's natural production of growth hormone (GH) and insulin-like growth factor-I (IGF-I). Because of its effective dual action, it's an advanced growth hormone stimulating product that has been clinically proven to increase GH and IGF-I levels, often well above physiological levels (in one clinical study using GHboost for a six week period, GH levels

were increased from 0.2 to 7.4 – the normal range was from 0 to 4). The increase in both GH and IGF-1 greatly enhances muscle development, strength, and size while decreasing bodyfat.

Used together, TestoBoost and GHboost maximize endogenous production of and maximize the anabolic and fat burning effects of testosterone, growth hormone and IGF-1.

- **NitAbol** – Grow muscles and burn bodyfat while you sleep. For information on NitAbol, see Appendix One.

Summary Of Supplements To Use

- General Supplements
- Supplements before, during and after training
- Myosin Protein during the day
- Nighttime Protein at night
- MRP LoCarb, LoCarb Sports Bar
- Creatine Advantage

Myosin And Nighttime Proteins

- Combination of whey, egg, soy and casein for spikes and long term elevation of amino acids
- Nighttime protein giving 2 spikes of amino acids for anabolic effect on protein synthesis, and increased basal elevations of protein all night for an anticatabolic effect.

Creatine Advantage

- Keeps the energy system in high gear despite the decreased caloric intake.
- Increases immediate energy levels through increasing PC levels – replenishing ATP. And by increasing glycolysis and increasing anapleurotic flux.

Cutting Phase

The purpose of this training phase is to decrease subcutaneous bodyfat while at the same time keeping as much muscle mass as we can. For bodybuilders this is the phase in which they get ripped and ready for competition. For recreational bodybuilders this is the phase in which they get buffed, and show as much visible muscle as possible. Although it's unlikely that you will get any significant amount of muscle hypertrophy, you can still get some increase in muscle size secondary to the increased vascularity of the muscle tissue.

Training in the Cutting Phase

In this phase we use what most people consider a more typical bodybuilding routine, using a variety of exercises designed to work both the large and small muscle groups. If done right, you can actually increase muscle size because of increased vascularity.

While you still make use of compound movements such as the squat, flat bench press, incline bench press, high pulls, deadlifts, bent over rowing, lat pulldowns and chins, you also make use of a variety of other movements meant to isolate one or more muscle groups or body parts. These movements included a variety of forearm and biceps curls and triceps presses, isolation exercises for the hamstrings, quads, calves, abdominal work, and a variety of isolation exercises for the shoulders, chest, and upper and lower back.

Since the main emphasis it to increase muscle metabolism and vascularity, you use lighter weights, beginning at least 30% less than the weights used in the strength phase, at doubling to tripling the repetitions in each set.

While the objective is still to fatigue the muscles completely in every set the emphasis is on doing this with lighter weights and more repetitions than in the Mass Phase. In the transition between the Strength Phases and the Cutting Phase you simply decrease the weight by 30% and double the reps.

In this phase the training sets up the conditions for consolidating muscle mass and decreasing bodyfat, while the diet meets the specific energy and macronutrient needs of this phase. As in the Mass and Strength Phases, in order to work the muscles adequately, especially as the weeks go by, you may have to use some special techniques, including partner assisted reps (usually for only one or two reps maximum), forced and partial reps, slow movements, negatives or eccentric training, super sets, etc.

Because you need less rest between sets, workout time in the Cutting Phase is usually about an hour, although doing some cardio will increase it. As well, you need to train more often, usually at least 4 days a week and up to twice a day, since you are trying to attain a thermogenic and vascular response from the training, and need less time to recover from the workouts.

It's a good idea to do split workouts during the Cutting Phase. That is you only concentrate of a limited number of muscle groups per day, covering all of the muscle groups once to twice, and sometimes even three times a week. For example a classic six day split, which covers each muscle group twice a week, would work legs, calves and shoulders on day one, chest and biceps on day two, back and triceps on day three, legs, calves and shoulders on day four, chest and biceps on day six and day 7 would be a rest day.

Another example is a 5-day split routine that works one muscle group each day: You should do four to five sets of each exercise with the reps should be in the 12 to 20 range depending on the exercise.

Day One (Chest)	Day Two (Back)
➲ Bench Press ➲ Dumbbell Flyes ➲ Cable Cross Overs	➲ Bent Over Rows ➲ T-Bar Rows ➲ Lat Pulldowns ➲ Seated Cable Rows
Day Three (Shoulders)	**Day Four (Arms)**
➲ Military Press ➲ Dumbbell Presses ➲ Dumbbell Side Laterals ➲ Bentover Dumbbell Laterals ➲ Dumbbell Shrugs	➲ Barbell Curls ➲ Dumbbell Curls ➲ Concentration Curls ➲ Triceps Extensions ➲ Seated Dumbbell Extensions ➲ Seated Barbell Extensions
Day Five (Legs)	
➲ Squats ➲ Leg Curls ➲ Leg Extensions ➲ Standing Calf Raises ➲ Seated Calf Raises	

Ab workout is done daily at end of workout. Also can do cardio for 15-45 minutes each day.

Duration of the Cutting Phase

The length of the Cutting Phase can vary widely, depending on how much fat you have to lose and how fast you want to take it off. Ideally the cutting phase can last anywhere from 8 to 16 weeks.

Nutrition for the Cutting Phase

During this phase, the classical cutting or definition phase, we go through the process of decreasing weight and bodyfat to whatever level is needed, while at the same time maintaining muscle mass.

The nutrition goals in the Cutting Phase is to maintain as much of the muscle mass as possible while decreasing bodyfat levels to the single digits.

Again, we do not change the mechanics of the Metabolic Diet in any phase, at least as far as the carb intakes. It's always 5 to 6 days high protein, low followed by 24-48 hours of carb loading. The only thing we change is the amount of calories and fat we eat. Since it's important to keep protein levels high (perhaps even higher than when in the other phases since as you lower calories, more protein is oxidized directly for energy, and used to form glucose through the gluconeogenesis) and carbs are already low, we have to decrease the amount of fat we eat during the low carb phase and to a lesser extent through the higher carb phase.

In the Cutting or Definition Phase we will be cutting calories as a way of trimming fat off the body. The reason we can do this is quite simple. We have trained our bodies to burn fat as its primary fuel, so as we decrease the caloric intake and dietary fat levels, the body naturally turns to using our bodyfat as fuel and continues to spare muscle.

Lower Dietary Fat When Fat Adapted

- Once fat adapted and you are into the Cutting Phase the amount of fat in the diet naturally decreases. The body then uses breaks down and uses bodyfat as its primary fuel.
- Thus you cut back on only dietary fat as you drop calories.
- **Protein intake stays the same or increases. You need to keep protein levels as high or higher than the Mass Phase since some protein now oxidized for fuel. This protein should come from dietary intake and thus spare muscle.**

As a rule of thumb, you should cut 500 calories a day from your diet the first week. If you were at say 4,000 during the Strength Phase cut it to 3,500 per day during the first week of your cutting. The next week you should drop another 200 to 500 from the daily diet, depending on how many calories you are taking in. For example someone taking in only 2000 calories would only cut down 200 calories. During this time you must measure bodyfat weekly. What you want to do is LOSE ROUGHLY 1.5-2 POUNDS OR 0.7 TO 1 KG OF BODYFAT EACH WEEK. Losing this amount of weight a week will insure that you do not lose appreciable lean mass as you cut.

If you find at the end of the second week that you have lost less than 1.5 pounds during the week, you will know you should cut another 200 to 500 calories the next week and continue cutting calories in subsequent weeks, anywhere from 100 to 500 calories until you are at the 1.5 level. Likewise, if you are losing more than 2 pounds of bodyfat during the week you will know you have cut too many calories and will need to adjust them upward.

And you do not have to make the cuts in specific calorie increments. You can fine tune how many calories you add or subtract in any amount. The usual progression is to make the changes 500 calories at a time the first time, and then maybe 100 to 500 calories the next few weeks and then 100 to 200 calories at a time as you get closer to your goal.

The important thing to remember here is that it's not calories we are really after. It's bodyfat. Because of this you have got to allow for individual variations in calorie count to get that optimum 1.5 to 2 pounds of fat loss. You will be doing plenty of experimentation in this phase to find the right caloric intake for you. Though the 500 calorie drops we outlined above seem to be a good general starting point, especially for those starting with the higher calorie intakes, you are going to have to find what works best for you. Also the calorie levels you eventually drop to will vary according to your initial caloric intake as well as to you metabolism and how you respond to the calorie cuts.

For example, I have dropped some bodybuilders on the diet from a 5,000 calorie a day level to 3,000 in the cutting phase. In a few others, I have taken them as low as 1,500 to see what happens. If they are losing a fair amount of bodyfat (remember the 1.5-2 pound guideline), getting leaner and not losing significant lean body mass I will leave them at that level until they "lean out". At that point, I will increase calories gradually to the point that they will maintain or possibly even lose bodyfat while increasing lean mass again.

Bodybuilders who just want to cut up and are starting at a higher bodyfat level can go directly into the Cutting Phase. They should start at a reasonable daily calorie value, usually15 CALORIES PER POUND OR 33 CALORIES PER KG OF BODYWEIGHT. Someone weighing 200 lbs, 0r 91 Kg, at say 17% bodyfat should start at around 3000 calories a day and then follow the instructions above on calorie adjustments needed to maintain the optimum weekly fat loss and minimal loss of muscle mass.

Be sure that you do not start too low. You will have plenty of time to lose that bodyfat in the right way. If you start too low the lack of food may be more of a problem than the lack of carbs, and may sabotage your efforts to stick to the diet through the all-important first week.

Keys To Success In The Cutting Phase

1. Measure bodyfat weekly
2. Lose 1.5-2 pounds (.7 to 1 Kg) a week
3. Experiment with caloric intake. Cutting 500 per day the first week and 100-500 per day in subsequent weeks is a rough guideline
4. Refine your contest preparation
5. Experiment with foods

Experiment With Foods

Basically, the Metabolic Diet's "5-day, 2-day" week is almost like getting a person in shape for a contest every week. In the weekend carb loading part of the diet, you will find out exactly how many hours you can load up on carbs before you begin to smooth out and lose your contest look.

When you get to your Pre-Contest Phase you really will not have to make many changes. You will be doing the same thing you have been doing for the last several weeks in the Cutting Phase. You will go off the higher fat, high protein diet and carb up to dramatically increase the glycogen and water inside the muscle cell. You want them swollen and big but you will cut off the carbs before you begin to reservoir extra-cellular water or fat and smooth out.

During the Cutting Phase, you will also want to be refining contest preparation. Play with the kinds of foods you eat on the weekends to see what gives you maximum muscle size. You will know on Monday morning if what you have been eating is right for you. If it is, you will be looking good. Muscles will be huge and you will be cut up with a nice, pronounced vascularity.

If you do not look good, you will know you did something wrong. Go back and rework your diet the next weekend and see if you can get some improvement. That is the beauty of this diet. By the time a contest approaches, you have already perfected your contest diet by practicing it during the Cutting Phase.

On the old carb diet, you did this only once. On this diet you do it every week during the "cutting" phase and you become an expert in how to manipulate your body for a contest.
Experiment with high and low sugar foods and percentages of fat intake on these weekends. See what they do for you. Treat each weekend as if your contest were imminent. That way you will know what it takes to come into a contest looking your best. You will also

experience an increase in confidence because you will know what to expect from your body and how to get it contest ready.

Supplements for the Cutting Phase

Cycling nutritional supplements means using those supplements that are phase specific so that a different set of supplements is used in each phase. As well, supplements should be taken at the rights times and for the right reasons.

Because of the different demands that each phase of training puts on the body, there are different needs to satisfy when talking about diet and nutritional supplements. For example, there are vast differences in dietary needs and the effects of various supplements between the mass and definition phases.

As well, there are differences in nutritional supplements used on days that you train and on rest days. Manipulating the diet and nutritional supplement use in and around training increases the anabolic and fat burning effects of the training and can decrease recuperation time and your abilities to perform at the next training session.

The different kinds of training that are followed in say the mass and cutting phases require specific dietary modifications and the use of different nutritional supplements. Other variables that also impact on the kind of diet followed and nutritional supplements used include the bodybuilders training background and the level that he or she has reached. Novice bodybuilders, in which the gains come relatively easy even with simple training routines and a diet high in calories and protein, do not need the sophisticated dietary modifications and cutting edge nutritional supplements that are a must if the more advanced bodybuilder is to improve.

In the Definition or Cutting Phase the supplements come into their own and are extremely useful in maintaining and raising the anabolic and fat burning response to the Metabolic Diet and training. That is because you are having to consistently cut calories so that your body effectively uses your bodyfat as fuel. In so doing, your system tends to change your hormones and metabolism to a survivalist mode, one that is counter productive to our goals, to maximize muscle mass while at the same time minimizing bodyfat. The Metabolic Diet is a big help here but the supplements are also important.

- **Exersol**, consisting of **Resolve**, **Power Drink** and **Amino**, works synergistically with the Metabolic Diet to help you reach your goals faster and more effectively.
- **The LoCarb MRP** and **LoCarb Sports Bars**, because of their complete nutritional makeup, can be used as meal substitutes or snacks and will be a big help when cutting calories. See above for more details.

- **Creatine Advantage** keeps the energy system in high gear despite the decreased caloric intake. Added amino acids and dipeptides allow a natural increase in the absorption and utilization of creatine and increase the volumizing, anticatabolic and anabolic effect of the formula. The added energy ingredients make Creatine Advantage the most advanced creatine and energy mix, one that will maximize energy, muscle mass and performance.

- **Metabolic** can really make the difference by counteracting the effects of the low calorie diet on the thyroid, adrenal and hormonal functions of the body. Metabolic optimizes the effects of thyroid hormone, decreases cortisone levels, naturally increases levels of growth hormone and testosterone (in both men and women), and increases the body's natural insulin sensitivity. These effects increase weight and fat loss while maintaining or even increasing muscle mass.

- **Myosin** Protein allows you to keep protein levels up at a time when it might be difficult to take in enough protein from foods while at the same time cutting calories. Myosin Protein Complex is an advanced synergistic blend of high quality protein powders, combining both fast and slow proteins, and including a specially developed source of glutamine peptides.

- **TestoBoost** contains several natural ingredients and is designed to improve natural testosterone formation, and decrease any potential side effects from conversion of testosterone to estrogens and dihydrotestosterone. By boosting the body's natural testosterone, TestoBoost increases muscle mass, decreases bodyfat and increases sexual desire.

- **GHboost** is formulated to increase muscle mass and decrease bodyfat by enhancing the body's natural production of growth hormone (GH) and insulin-like growth factor-I (IGF-I). Because of its effective dual action, it's an advanced growth hormone stimulating product that has been clinically proven to increase GH and IGF-I levels, often well above physiological levels (in one clinical study using GHboost for a six week period, GH levels were increased from 0.2 to 7.4 – the normal range was from 0 to 4). The increase in both GH and IGF-1 greatly enhances muscle development, strength, and size while decreasing bodyfat.

Used together, TestoBoost and GHboost maximize endogenous production of and maximize the anabolic and fat burning effects of testosterone, growth hormone and IGF-1. These two supplements counteract the normal decline in these hormones seen in calorie restricted diets.
NitAbol is another combination formulation to my nutritional supplement lineup. This combo is especially useful in the Cutting Phase as it counteracts the loss of muscle mass and increases fat loss during sleep.

NitAbol is a precise combination of proteins and amino acids which has a maximum effect on stimulating protein synthesis, maximizing testosterone, growth hormone, IGF-1 and the anabolic effects of insulin, decreasing bodyfat, and stimulating the recovery, **All while you sleep**.

The Pre-Contest Phase

One of the many advantages of this diet is that, if you want to enter a lot of contests, you can manipulate your diet so you never get much above the 8 percent bodyfat level. You do not have those huge gains in bodyfat here. At 8 percent, you can drop to contest level in 2-3 weeks. It will not take a great deal of time.

Still, for most purposes you will want to go into the Pre-contest Phase of diet and training about 16 weeks before a major contest to get ready. Again, because you already know what you need to do from previous weekends on the diet, you will only be doing some fine tuning here by lowering and increasing calories a bit as needed. You shouldn't be doing anything much out of the ordinary.

By the final 6-8 weeks before the contest you should look fairly close to how you want to be on stage. With this diet you can control things so you know exactly where you are at each week. Following the weekend carb loading portion of your diet you should be looking great on Monday, ready to hit the gym hard with the high glycogen levels, muscle swelling and other benefits to be derived by a well-honed weekend diet strategy.

Panic Attacks

One of the things bodybuilders do to sabotage themselves before contests is to panic. They will find themselves too fat and begin doing aerobics thinking this will get the extra bodyfat off for them. At a minimum, doing about a half hour of aerobics consistently is not going to harm you. You will burn up more free fatty acids than you would not doing enough work and this will take off some bodyfat and get you closer to your goals.

But bodybuilders begin to panic and overdo it. They will start doing 3-4 hours a day of aerobics to get that fat off and all they do is exhaust energy stores so that the body starts using its own muscle tissue for energy. Obviously, this is not what you want to do so close to a contest.
Likewise, if you are really in trouble you can start pigging out to build mass while thinking that aerobics will make up for the fat buildup. It's not going to work. Increasing calories and aerobics will most probably just increase catabolic activity in your body.

Aerobics, while burning fat, can also destroy muscle. Even if it doesn't do appreciable damage, it will still limit the amount of muscle you can put on to some degree. As a rule, the less calories you take in and the more time you allow yourself to lose the bodyfat, the less aerobics you will need to do and the more lean body mass you will retain. You need to allow yourself time to lose the bodyfat and gauge yourself effectively as you move toward a contest.

That is one of the things this diet does so well. With the weekend portion of the diet you will learn what foods to eat and how much to make yourself successful. You will be better able to track your progress and know what you will need to do for the contest beforehand. There will be no need for those rash decisions that throw a curve ball at your metabolism.

Messing Up A Good Thing

Above all, you want to make a smooth landing into a contest. You shouldn't be doing anything out of the ordinary. You certainly do not want to panic.

But some bodybuilders, in full control of their senses, will decide to try something new just before a contest. They are looking to get that final edge. They mess up. Their water table increases. They start with the sodium depletion or sodium loading trick. They will let loose with all sorts of things they have never tried before and all of a sudden they end up wondering how it was that they were looking so great and now look so bad.

Again, do not shock your system before a contest. Make a smooth landing into it. Do not throw everything away by trying to get the extra edge through some crazy stunt.

Fluid Retention

If you do tend to retain fluid, begin to restrict yourself to distilled water and low levels of sodium 24 hours before the competition. Also increase your potassium, magnesium and calcium intake.

Actually, most people tend to retain some fluid so these suggestions should be considered by all bodybuilders. You want as little extracellular fluid as possible to avoid smoothing out. On the other hand, intracellular fluid will increase cell size so you will be bigger. It also aids vascularity.

Distilled water and low sodium will serve to lower the extracellular fluid. Potassium will increase the amount of fluid inside the cell. Higher potassium levels are also better for muscle contractions though you want to be sure not to create potassium levels that are too high. Calcium, and magnesium, are important in avoiding cramping.

Do Not Overdo It

As we discussed above, you can go through the Pre-Contest Phase in preparation for a contest several times a year as long as you keep your fat levels lower. In this way, it really doesn't take much time to get into contest shape.

That being said, I'd suggest that you only got through the Pre-Contest Phase 4 times a year. That means a maximum of 4 contests a year. More than this is self defeating because I do not believe you will have the time to go back into the mass phase and use it properly.

You have got to go back and build up lean body mass to some extent between contests. This also means you will gain a bit of fat. You will still be bulking up and cutting down but it will not be like on the other diet where you bulk up so much that you gain so much bodyfat that by the time you lose it you are no better off than when you started.

Again, the goal here is to make you bigger, stronger and more cut from contest to contest and year-to-year. That is what the Metabolic Diet is all about.

1-2 Weeks Out

You should stop training 1-2 weeks out from the contest. That is pretty standard wherever you go. My advice is to do your last heavy training session 10 days before the contest. This will give your muscles maximum time to recuperate and achieve maximum growth. Do not worry about maintaining muscle mass and tone. The posing you will be doing will take care of that and also give you some aerobic activity. Posing should, of course, be continued throughout this entire period, with the exception of the day before the contest.

But though you will shut down training heavy 10 days or so before a contest, this is the only time you should back off. Some people think that just because they are on the Metabolic Diet, they do not have to work as hard. That is simply not true. All you are going to do by cutting back in training is limit the effectiveness of the diet and your ultimate growth.

The two, diet and training, work hand in hand. Exercise actually complements the Metabolic Diet. Hormonal changes caused by exercise result in an increase in the activity of the enzyme lipoprotein lipase (LPL) in the muscle. This in turn causes increased use of free fatty acids and decreases fat buildup.

We will cover some more about what kind of exercise is best in concert with the Metabolic Diet in a later addendum. For now, suffice it to say that both training and lifestyle work hand in hand with the Metabolic Diet in maximizing its benefits.

Countdown To Contest

Above we talked about the importance of experimenting with carb loading duration and foods to learn when and how your body looks its best. That is basically the trick in perfecting that critical contest diet.

During the weekend carb loading part of the diet you note how many hours into it that you look your very best. You refine that time by experimenting with the types of food you eat to precisely dial in that time when you are at your best so you can use this information when the contest arrives.

What you will eventually find is that there is a day in the week when you will look your very best. All the water you have gained during your carb load will be drained out and you will have just the right balance between glycogen in the muscle and water to look your best. You will feel great, too. Some people will look their best on Monday. Some on Tuesday. Some on Wednesday. Everybody's system works differently and you will find wide differences here. The goal is to find the right day FOR YOU, that day when you are at your best consistently, each week.

Most contests come on Saturday. Suppose you have found that you look your best on Wednesday of each week. Your goal then is to basically make the Saturday of your contest like a Wednesday. Because you look your best 3 days after your carb load, you want to complete a carb loading 3 days before the contest to make sure you look your best. Therefore, the Tuesday and Wednesday before the contest you carb up so that 3 days later, on Saturday, you will look your best.

An important point here is that, the weekend before the contest, you will not carb up as usual. To carb up on the weekend and then carb up again two or three days later may well spill you back over to a carb-burning metabolism and smooth you out for that Saturday contest. Because of this you skip your carb load the weekend before a contest. That way you will be on the high protein, higher fat part of the Metabolic Diet for 8 straight days, from the Monday 2 weeks before the contest to the Tuesday before the contest. At that point you will begin your pre-contest carb load so you will hit the contest just right.
This is one area where the Metabolic Diet has a big advantage over the competition. When you are on the high carb diet you are basically always carbing up so it's difficult to manipulate the diet so the body will respond well to your carb loading attempt before the contest.

What often happens is that you will get off your high carb diet for 3 days at the beginning of the week before a competition and go low carb for 72 hours. Then you will carb up to try and hit the contest right. The problem is, you really do not know how your body's going to react. Everything could work out well. Then again, you could experience a complete disaster.

It's Russian roulette. You have got maybe a 50 percent chance of hitting the mark. Here you have maybe had a year to prepare for the contest. You have been disciplined and dedicated. Yet you miss the mark when you hit the stage because of the uncertainty of the high carb diet.

With the Metabolic Diet, you will know the exact hour when you look your best. Your body's going through the cycle every week. It's become predictable and consistent. You will be dialed in and know what to expect. You will not be doing anything different than you have done in the preceding months.

KEYS TO SUCCESS IN THE PRE-CONTEST PHASE

1. Begin this phase 16 weeks before contest
2. By 6-8 weeks out you should be close to your contest look
3. Do not panic or make rash decisions
4. Stick with the program
5. Do not overdo aerobics
6. Stop training 1-2 weeks out
7. Skip your carb load the weekend before the contest
8. Time your carb load so you will look your best at prejudging
9. Allow a 4-hour "fail-safe" period
10. Begin to drink distilled water, increase potassium, magnesium and calcium, and reduce sodium 24 hours before contest
11. Be careful with diet after prejudging

Prejudging

You will want that exact hour when you look your best to coincide with prejudging. This is where most decisions are made and this is where you will want to look your absolute best.

But the body is not a perfectly predictable instrument. That is why, to make sure you do not smooth out, you will want to give yourself 4 hours of extra time as a kind of "fail-safe" mechanism for prejudging.

So, if you find you are at your best 48 hours after carb loading and prejudging will take place at 2:00 on Saturday, count back 48 hours. This will put you at 2:00 Thursday. Give yourself the extra four hours mentioned above and you will find yourself completing carb loading at 6:00 P.M. on Thursday.

You will also want to look good at the evening show, especially if judging is close and will be ultimately decided in the evening. Fortunately, you have usually got a window, a several hour period, where you look good and that will carry over to the evening session.

Still, you have got to be careful. Some competitors will look great for prejudging and then go out and eat thinking it's all over. They will come in bloated and retaining water for the evening show and, in a close competition, lose out because of it. You have got to stay tight all day. Keep diet minimal and in the higher fat mode. Even having food in your stomach will create a slight bulge. You want to keep everything nice and flat so keep your regimen going through the evening contest.

The above is, of course, just an example. You will have to work with the diet to find the best approach for you. The big difference between this diet and whatever you have been on before is the precision with which you can plan your contest regimen. Not only does the Metabolic Diet build muscle and burn fat, it also gives you a weekly opportunity to practice and prepare for a contest so you can manipulate your diet to the very best effect.

No more 48 hour carb loads before a contest. No more uncertainty or panic. The Metabolic Diet lets you to know exactly what you need to do to look your best well before the actual competition takes place.

Supplements for the Pre-Contest Phase

There is not much of a difference in the supplements you use in the Cutting and Pre-Contest Phases. The only thing to watch out for is the effects some of the supplements may have on your definition. For example some bodybuilders discontinue creatine a few weeks out from the competition because they retain more water and less defined if they stay on it. Also the use of certain supplements, such as **Myosin Protein**, **Metabolic** (to optimize the hormones including insulin, thyroid), **ReNew** (useful for overtraining or if you are getting run down) and **JointSupport** (for preventing and treating injuries and overtraining), usually increases as the competition gets closer.

Rest Phase

While we are discussing the Cutting Phase it's a good idea to cover the Rest Phase that normally follows. The Rest Phase is ideally a period of time in which you chill out, cut back on your training and get yourself mentally and physically "healed" for the next push. In the Rest Phase it's also a good idea to relax your diet and cut back on your nutritional supplement use. Basically give your mind and body a change to get back to normal, away from the self imposed rigors and schedules. The Rest Phase may even be a time during which you simply gave up training for a period of time for one reason or another.

Nutrition for the Rest Phase (Post Contest or Break)

During the Rest Phase I usually suggest going off the strict part of the Metabolic Diet and reintroducing a moderate amount of carbs, anywhere from 20 to 50%, cutting back on the protein and going on a moderate fat diet. In other words you are following a diet that is pretty close to the normal North American Diet.

And do not worry about having problems getting strict with the Metabolic Diet when it's time. Your body will "remember" and it will be much easier to get back in the grove.

Nutritional Supplements for the Rest Phase

Again, during the Rest Phase back off on all your supplements except maybe MVM, the vitamin and mineral supplement. The one other supplement you may want to use during this phase is **ReNew** since this supplement is meant to get your system, and especially your immune system, back to normal.

ReNew™...Advanced Immune System Enhancer

ReNew is formulated not only to enhance the immune system, but also to normalize the metabolism and to naturally support thyroid, testosterone, GH, insulin and andrenergic function. It's the perfect nutritional supplement to deal with workout fatigue and at the end of a long periodization session.

Your immune system is the first line of defense against stress, whether physical or emotional. ReNew can naturally boost your immunity by providing the necessary nutritional building blocks for enhancing and supporting the immune system. As such, ReNew is useful for optimizing muscle recovery, and reducing the effects of excessive exercise.

For Additional Product Information, FAQs, Sample Diets, Calorie and Carb Charts, Training Information and Routines, Articles and much more, visit www.MetabolicDiet.com and www.CoachSOS.com, and soon www.AnabolicSolution.com, on a regular basis.

APPENDIX ONE

Cellusol 1-2-3 System

The Complete Nutritional Supplement Cellulite and Weight Loss Solution

Cellusol is a multi phase supplement and by far the most advanced weight and fat loss formula ever. It's light years ahead of anything out there right now including prescription diet aids. Cellusol has more than ten times the active ingredients of any other weight loss product, and instead of using one or two approaches, like most other products, it attacks the problems of weight and fat loss from several directions ensuring both immediate, and more importantly, long-term success.

Cellusol has been formulated to accomplish maximum weight and fat loss, **especially cellulite**, while at the same time minimizing the loss of muscle. This means that the weight you lose will be mostly bodyfat and you will look both fit and trim as you lose your weight.

Cellusol is a stacked/cycled product consisting of 3 formulations. Each formulation is meant to attack the problem of maximizing body composition from a different angle. For example for the first two weeks

For the first two weeks you take Thermo. Thermo increases metabolic rate and as such increases energy output, plus it increases the breakdown and burning off of bodyfat, including cellulite, and help maintain muscle.

For the next two weeks it's Metabolic, which is meant to help you keep your precious muscle and keep the fat coming off. It also optimizes the important hormones and processes in your body including increasing insulin sensitivity, and regulating growth hormone, testosterone and thyroid levels.

For the next two weeks it's Renew, a sophisticated, cutting edge product meant to enhance the immune systems and support your metabolism – essentially to get the body raring to go and ready for the weight and fat loss actions of Thermo.

Each package of Cellusol contains enough product for two successive cycles – each 6-week cycle will take you to a new level of weight and fat loss. By cycling each formula for a two-week period you will not allow your body to adapt to any one formula and as such your weight and fat loss will not plateau. You will continue to lose weight and bodyfat in each of the six-week cycles.

Because one of the phases is a renewal phase, during each six-week cycle you will be allowing your body to regain it's normal balance and become more receptive to the weight and fat loss supplements that are in the other two formulations. You will no longer have to worry about staying on any supplement for too long and reaching a weight and fat loss plateau because your body gets used to the supplements, or go through a rebound and gain your weight back when you stop taking the weight loss aids.

While Cellusol will work it's magic alone, it works best if you follow a complete exercise and nutrition program. Regular exercise and going on the Metabolic Diet will maximize Cellusol's effects on body composition and weight and fat loss and allow you to reach your goals much faster and easier. The end result of using all three will be a fit and toned body that you will be proud of.

- Phase One Formulation – Thermo
- Phase Two Formulation – Metabolic
- Phase Three Formulation – ReNew

Thermo – Advanced Thermogenic and Anabolic Formula

Thermo is formulated to increase energy levels for training, maximize fat loss by increasing fat oxidation and decreasing fat deposition, while at the same time maintaining muscle mass.
Thermo increases the body's thermogenic response, increases energy for training, has anticatabolic and anabolic properties that maintains muscle mass, increases fat breakdown and fatty acid utilization, decreases appetite, increases insulin sensitivity and supports thyroid hormone activity.

Metabolic – Advanced Anabolic and Fat Loss Primer

Metabolic is formulated to optimize the body's hormones in order to maximize the anabolic and fat burning effects of exercise.
Metabolic optimizes the effects of thyroid hormone, decreases cortisone levels and increases levels of growth hormone and testosterone (in both men and women) along with increasing insulin sensitivity. These effects increase weight and fat loss while maintaining or even increasing muscle mass. As well, the hormonal environment created by Metabolic will allow cellulite, that stubborn dimpled fat, to be oxidized along with the rest of the bodyfat.

ReNew – Homeostatic and Immune System Enhancer

ReNew is a premier product that, as part of the Cellusol team, enhances and stabilizes weight and fat loss and allows the body to return to an optimal metabolic and immune state where it's once again ready and able to respond to the next two Cellusol cycles. With ReNew you return to a state where the body solidifies previous weight and fat losses and is once again sensitive and responsive to both Thermo and Metabolic. In a sense, ReNew rejuvenates your body so that it is ready and able to make dramatic weight and fat losses.

Exersol 1-2-3 System

The Complete Exercise Solution

Resolve	Power Drink	Amino

Exersol Competition

Resolve	Competition	Power Drink	Amino

Exersol is a three-phase exercise-oriented nutritional support system that takes the guesswork out of what supplements to use before, during and after training. As the most scientifically advanced and sophisticated exercise orientated nutritional support system ever formulated, its use is invaluable for anyone who wants to lose bodyfat and build muscle.

Exersol is the Complete Nutritional Supplement Training Solution and as such, you have the peace of mind that comes with knowing you have everything you could possibly ever need to maximize the anabolic and fat burning effects of exercise. You also have the peace of mind knowing that there is absolutely nothing out there that even comes close to doing what Exersol will do for your training and body composition, regardless of price, reputation and claims.

Exersol has been formulated to allow you to get the most from your training efforts. Not only will it maximize the fat burning and muscle building effects of exercise but it will allow you to train longer, harder and more effectively, and make the training you do much more productive.

- Formula Number One – Either Resolve or Resolve Competition before Training
- Formula Number Two – Power Drink – During Training
- Formula Number Three – Amino – After Training

Resolve and Resolve Competition –

Advanced Pre-Workout Anabolic and Fat Burning Primers

Resolve and Resolve Competition are the ultimate pre training formulations. They prime your metabolism so your body can optimize the anabolic and fat burning effects of exercise.

These formulas will provide anticatabolic and anabolic effects by increasing levels of testosterone and growth hormone, decreasing protein breakdown, increasing protein synthesis and providing cell volumizing effects that increase muscle growth. They also maximize ATP and phosphocreatine (PC) functioning, as well as gluconeogenic and other processes, allowing for more strength and stamina. As well, it provides potent thermogenic and fat loss properties, increasing fat breakdown and utilization and decreasing fat buildup. And finally they exert a potent antioxidant effect to decrease muscle tissue injury and soreness.

While almost everyone considers post training nutrition as being important, many fail to realize that the intake of amino acids and other ingredients prior to training is as, or perhaps even more important for maximizing the anabolic and fat burning response to exercise.

Resolve and Resolve Competition, by increasing lipolysis, and thus the availability of fatty acids, complement the Metabolic Diet, which increases fat oxidation. The combination of increased bodyfat breakdown and increased burning of fat for energy make Resolve and Resolve Competition ideal pre-workout primers for those on the Metabolic Diet. As well, Resolve and Resolve Competition contain no carbohydrates.

Resolve – with ephedrine and yohimbine

- Maximizes muscle growth and strength and minimizes bodyfat
- Optimizes the anabolic and fat burning effects of exercise
- Decreases muscle breakdown and increases protein synthesis

Resolve Competition – with no ephedrine or yohimbine but with neurotransmitter precursors

- Maximizes the muscle building and fat burning effects of exercise
- Optimizes your metabolism
- Supplies increased energy for training even though it's stimulant and ephedrine free

Power Drink

Advanced Anabolic Training Drink

Power Drink is a revolutionary new concept in training drinks. There is nothing even close to it on the market. This drink provides the nutrients necessary to maximize muscle mass by increasing the anabolic and decreasing the catabolic effects of exercise, and increasing the mobilization and oxidation of bodyfat.

Power Drink contains over 30 grams of whey protein isolate (a "fast" protein that results in high systemic amino acid levels), which is over 25% branched chain amino acids. As well, the formula contains several amino acids (arginine, alanine, taurine), glutamine peptides, creatine, ribose, electrolytes and other ingredients that will replace and replenish nutrients and fluid lost through exercise, prevent muscle cramps, and increase training time and efficiency.

The formula contains no carbohydrates or fat except for glycerol (which does not raise either glucose or insulin levels appreciably, and ribose, which increases the reformation of ATP and other important cellular compounds).

- Maximizes training energy and efficiency
- Increases training effort and energy
- Maximizes muscle mass and increases fat oxidation

Amino

Complete Amino Acid Formula

Amino, the cutting-edge amino acid formulation, maximizes protein synthesis by providing you with a quick and potent boost of anabolic and anticatabolic amino acids. The high systemic levels of important amino acids provided by Amino has a direct potent effect on protein synthesis, and at the same time increases systemic levels of the potent anabolic hormones, including insulin, testosterone and growth hormone.

Used immediately after training it's an easy to take, easy on the stomach, source of amino acids that kicks protein synthesis into high gear so you can begin taking advantage of that post-training window of opportunity. Amino is formulated to provide a square wave increase in the availability of blood amino acids within minutes after ingestion, and a measurable increase in muscle protein synthesis within less than half an hour – much faster than other post exercise supplements.

Amino is an enhanced, cutting-edge amino acid formula consisting of free amino acids, a hefty dose of special glutamine and other peptides, and several special ingredients. The amino acid, peptide blend, and special ingredients in Amino work together synergistically to immediately increase blood amino acid levels, insulin sensitivity and insulin levels, as well as growth hormone and testosterone levels, resulting in increased muscle protein synthesis which maximizes the anabolic and fat burning effects of exercise and combats overtraining.

Amino is the perfect supplement to take immediately after training since it provides an immediate anabolic effect with a minimum of gastrointestinal distress. It's also extremely useful throughout the day to give a rapid pulsed increase in amino acids and anabolic hormones that leads to short burst increases in muscle protein synthesis. Research has shown that pulses of high levels of amino acids is much more effective in increasing protein synthesis than sustained high levels.

- Maximizes protein synthesis after training and anytime it's used.
- Maximizes the anabolic and fat burning effects of exercise.
- Enhances recovery.

NitAbol

The Complete Night Time Anabolic/ Anticatabolic/Fat-Burning Combo

For Men and Women

INCREASE MUSCLE MASS AND DECREASE BODYFAT WHILE YOU SLEEP!

Goal of NitAbol is to counter the nighttime postabsorptive catabolic effects, increase recovery, fat burning and protein synthesis.

- Minimizes the catabolic effects of the postabsorptive phase
- Increases fat utilization over protein
- Increases insulin sensitivity
- Increases muscle, central nervous system and systemic recovery during sleep.
- Anti-inflammatory effects for increased recovery.

Three Products that make up NitAbol are:

- Myosin Protein Complex
- TestoBoost

- Ghboost

Myosin Protein Complex

Myosin Complex is the most advanced synergistic blend of the highest quality protein powders, peptides and amino acids on the market today, bar none. It contains the perfect amino acid mix to maximize protein synthesis, decrease muscle breakdown and enhance athletic performance.

GHboost

GHboost is formulated to increase muscle mass and decrease bodyfat by increasing the body's natural production of growth hormone (GH) and insulin-like growth factor-I (IGF-I). Because of its effective dual action, it's an advanced growth hormone stimulating product that has been clinically proven to increase GH and IGF-I levels, often well above physiological levels (in one clinical study using GHboost for a six week period, GH levels were increased from 0.2 to 7.4 – the normal range was from 0 to 4). The increase in both GH and IGF-I greatly enhances muscle development, strength, and size while decreasing bodyfat.

When used before bed it will increase the natural growth hormone spike associated with the first deep sleep cycle of the night (usually within 2 hours of going to sleep) and enhance the long term increase in insulin-like growth factor I (IGF-I). The combination increase of both hormones increases protein synthesis, decreases muscle catabolism, and increases the use of bodyfat as the main energy source all night long.

TestoBoost

TestoBoost maximizes your anabolic potential by physiologically elevating your natural testosterone levels. Not only does TestoBoost contain natural ingredients that increase testosterone formation, it also has ingredients that decrease any potential side effects from conversion of testosterone to estrogens and dihydrotestosterone. By boosting testosterone, TestoBoost has beneficial effects on increasing muscle mass, decreasing bodyfat, and on fertility and impotence.

TestoBoost is all natural and elevates serum testosterone levels without using any prohormones, compounds with potentially serious side effects and very little effects on testosterone levels.

Used at night TestoBoost adds to the anabolic and anticatabolic effects of GHboost to further increase protein synthesis, decrease muscle catabolism, enhance recovery and burn off bodyfat while you sleep.

Directions: For men: Four tablets before bed. For women: One tablet before bed.

Basics Behind NitAbol – The Night Time Stack**Goal –** To counter the nighttime post absorptive catabolic effects and increase recovery and protein synthesis.

Sleep dynamics different from when awake. But in Postabsorptive phase there is increased muscle catabolism especially in second half of sleep phase.
NitAbol Works by:

1. Minimizing the postabsorptive phase by modulating nutrient absorption and effects.
2. Increasing the use of fatty acids and decreasing the use of muscle protein (and thus decreasing muscle breakdown) for gluconeogenesis and oxidation as fuel.
3. Manipulating the anabolic and catabolic hormones to maximize protein synthesis and minimize protein breakdown during sleep.
4. Increasing cell hydration (volumizing) and as such stimulating protein synthesis.
5. Enhancing the Immune System to decrease catabolic cytokines and increase recovery.

Hormonal Manipulation With the Use of NitAbol

- Testosterone – increase
- Cortisol – decrease
- Growth Hormone – increase
- IGF-I – increase
- Insulin – increase amount and sensitivity
- Thyroid – control

Ingredients

Macronutrients

Combination of Proteins

Whey – fast protein – increase GH spike, Increase insulin.

- Casein – slow protein – delay postabsorptive phase.
- Milk Protein Isolate/Colostrum.
- Other proteins – egg, soy – decrease postabsorptive phase

Peptides and Amino Acids

Glutamine Peptides

- Branched Chain Amino Acids
- Glycine
- Arginine
- Lysine
- Ornithine

Carbohydrates

Not necessary as in significant amounts it will decrease GH and IGF-I secretion and the use of bodyfat as a primary fuel.

Micronutrients

Vitamins and Minerals

- Zinc – enhances testosterone synthesis
- Calcium & Magnesium
- Potassium – volumizing
- Sodium – volumizing
- Vitamins A, E – anticatabolic & antioxidant
- Vitamin A – increases insulin sensitivity

- Vitamin C – anticortisol and antioxidant

Additional Ingredients modify IGF-1, GH, Insulin, Testosterone, Cortisol, Thyroid, Glucagon, enhance Immune System, and decrease catabolic effects.

NitAbol Controls the Proinflammatory Cytokines

IL-1beta, IL-6, TNF-alpha that Produce a hypercatabolic state – net efflux of essential amino acids from skeletal muscle.

Ingredients to combat the Proinflammatory Cytokines include:

- Glutamine
- Ornithine
- Vitamin A and Vitamin E
- Whey, casein, soy proteins
- Milk Isolates
- Colostrum

EFA+

Essential Fatty Acid Formula

EFA+ is a multipurpose formulation designed to provide the full gamut of all the essential and conditionally essential fatty acids that are so important to optimizing your metabolism, maximizing the anabolic and fat-burning effects of exercise and dealing with minor muscle ache and joint pain after exercise.

EFAs are involved in:

- Hormone Production
- Muscle and Joint Tissue Repair
- Insulin Metabolism
- Fat Burning

Regular supplementation with EFA+ ensures essential and conditionally essential fatty acids, such as omega-6, omega-3, EPA, DHA, CLA, GLA, and ALA are available to support the optimal metabolic response to intense exercise. Antioxidants in EFA+ dramatically enhance the benefits of the EFAs.

With its many ingredients working in concert, EFA+:

- Optimizes metabolism to make the best use of the anabolic and fat burning effects of exercise.
- Improves testosterone production and increases growth hormone secretion
- Increases the breakdown and oxidation of bodyfat.
- Increases lean body mass.
- Improves natural insulin sensitivity.
- Supports the body's immune system.
- Decreases inflammation, muscle ache and joint pain secondary to excessive exercise.

BOTTOM LINE

If you exercise, you shouldn't be without EFA+ since it enhances fat loss, increases lean muscle mass, and allows you to train more effectively with fewer aches, pains and injuries.

Myosin Protein COMPLEX

Myosin Protein Complex is the most advanced, synergistic blend of the highest quality protein powders, peptides and amino acids on the market today, bar none. It contains the perfect amino acid mix to maximize protein synthesis, decrease muscle breakdown and enhance athletic performance.

We use a variety of the highest quality protein powder to make use of the special characteristics of each and thus enhancing their overall effect while at the same time eliminating their relative disadvantages. Because of the gentle processes used to isolate the various proteins, the formula maintains the beneficial immune and other effects of the undenatured whey, casein, egg and soy proteins.

Myosin Complex – (Soy protein isolate, egg protein, CFM whey protein isolate, whey protein hydrolysate, calcium/sodium caseinate, and glutamine peptides) combines both fast and slow proteins and peptides that flood the body with an initial large peaked pulse of amino acids and then a sustained release that maintains protein synthesis and decreases muscle breakdown for hours. For this reason Myosin Protein is especially useful as a night time protein, especially when used in combination with Ghboost and TestoBoost (all three make up my NitAbol combo).

The blend of proteins and amino acids in Myosin Protein is unique and contains the exact amino acid formulation to maximize protein synthesis and minimize protein breakdown. Myosin provides for a varied spectrum of blood amino acids with spikes from the whey protein, intermediate spikes from the egg and soy, and a prolonged amino acid response from the slowly absorbed casein. Myosin Protein was engineered to increase protein synthesis with spikes of blood amino acids and to decrease protein/muscle breakdown with a sustained low level increase in blood amino acids.

And you cannot compare even the most sophisticated whey protein with Myosin Protein. Myosin has all the advantages of the best whey protein on the market, and of all the other proteins, peptides and amino acids that make it up. This is because the body treats the mix of proteins as if each protein was taken separately. Thus these proteins, even when taken together, maintain their different (fast, intermediate and slow) absorption rates.

Myosin Protein is also engineered to increase protein synthesis by increasing the anabolic hormones (including insulin and GH thus complementing GHboost) and decreasing the catabolic ones, and by providing the body with an increased immune response to combat overtraining and maximize the anabolic and fat burning effects of exercise.

MRP LoCarb

The Ultimate Anabolic, AntiCatabolic, Fat Burning Meal Replacement Shake

MRP LoCarb is the highest quality, best tasting, most nutritionally complete meal replacement shake on the market today, bar none.

It is the ultimate low carbohydrate meal replacement powder. Unlike some products that only have two or more ingredients and call themselves meal replacements, and others that have more but are still inadequate, MRP LoCarb is an engineered food that contains the full gamut of macro and micronutrients and is truly an anabolic, anticatabolic, and fat burning, full featured meal replacement.

MRP LoCarb is a high protein/low carbohydrate/moderate fat meal replacement powder containing the most advanced protein blend on the market, healthy fats (mono, poly and some saturated fats along with lecithin and an essential fatty acid blend containing omega-3 and omega-6 fatty acids), soluble fiber, a complete balanced Vitamin and Mineral profile, and less than 6 grams of carbs per serving!

The protein blend in MRP LoCarb contains a synergistic blend of proteins and a specially developed source of glutamine peptides that was developed for Myosin Protein Complex. It's engineered to increase protein synthesis by increasing the anabolic hormones and decreasing the catabolic ones, and by providing the body with an increased immune response to combat overtraining and maximize the anabolic and fat burning effects of exercise.

MRP LoCarb, because it's a complete low carbohydrate meal replacement powder, can be used in confidence by anyone on the Metabolic Diet and any low carbohydrate diet plain including Atkins' and Protein Power. It's also useful for those on the Metabolic Diet higher carb plans, or other higher carb diets, because the level of carbs can be easily modified by mixing the powder with milk or juices instead of water or simply by adding carbs in the form of fruits or other carb sources including easily available maltodextrins.

The use of MRP LoCarb within a few hours of training increases the training response and protein synthesis, maximizes rebound macronutrient replenishment and improves recovery. The special blend of proteins in MRP LoCarb, like the Myosin Protein blend, maximizes protein synthesis and minimize protein breakdown for several hours.

Easy to prepare and use, our MRP LoCarb simplifies meal planning and can be taken in place of any meal, as an in between meal and/or before bed snack, and as a delayed post training meal

LoCarb Sports Bars

The Ultimate Anabolic, AntiCatabolic, Fat Burning Sports Bar

LoCarb Sports Bars are the highest quality, most nutritionally complete sports bars on the market today, bar none.

The LoCarb Sports Bars have the nutrition and advantages of the MRP LoCarb meal replacement powders in a convenient and delicious bar. The bars can be used post-workout, or as a snack anytime since they can be easily kept on hand by in your gym bag, desk drawer, purse, glove compartment etc.

LoCarb Bars, unlike high sugar and carb sport bars that flood today's marketplace, have a high protein and low carb content and are an ideal snack for people on The Metabolic Diet or who are watching their carb intake. And unlike the other locarb, high protein bars, LoCarb Sports Bars are nutritionally complete, with nutrients that will help you achieve your body composition goals.

The bottom line is that our LoCarb Sports Bars are the Ultimate High Protein/Low Carb Meal Replacement Bars on the market today. They have the most effective macronutrient and micronutrient content for maximizing the anabolic and fat loss effects of exercise.

ReNew

Advanced Recovery and Immune System Enhancer

ReNew is formulated not only to enhance the immune system, but also to normalize the metabolism, improve recovery, and to naturally support thyroid, testosterone, GH, insulin and the function of the adrenal glands.

It's the perfect nutritional supplement to deal with workout fatigue and to use at the end of a long periodization session.

Your immune system is the first line of defense against stress, whether physical or emotional. ReNew can naturally boost your immunity by providing the necessary nutritional building blocks for enhancing and supporting the immune system. As such, ReNew is useful for optimizing muscle recovery, and reducing the effects of excessive exercise.

ReNew is a premier product that is also part of the Cellusol team. It enhances and stabilizes weight and fat loss and allows the body to return to an optimal metabolic and immune state where it's once again ready and able to respond to the next two Cellusol cycles.

With ReNew you return to a state where the body solidifies previous weight and fat losses and is once again sensitive and responsive to both Thermo and Metabolic. In a sense, ReNew rejuvenates your body so that it is ready and able to make dramatic weight and fat losses.

Regulate

Regulate is an potent blend of natural soluble and insoluble fibers, plus probiotic ingredients, formulated for both preventing and treating constipation, frequent bowel movements, and other problems.

Regulate, by delaying gastric emptying and reducing the time to perceived fullness, is effective as an appetite suppressant. Taken before meals or whenever hungry, Regulate lessens your hunger and curbs cravings.

The various soluble fibers and other compounds contained in Regulate have also been found useful to:

- Maintain cholesterol levels that are already within normal range.
- Support a healthy heart.
- Increase natural insulin sensitivity.
- Has probiotic effects – promotes growth of beneficial bacteria in bowels.
- Constipation – especially recommended in the initial stages of the Metabolic Diet.
- Frequent bowel movements.
- Other bowel problems including hemorrhoids, irritable bowel syndrome, and inflammatory colitis (ulcerative colitis, Crohn's disease, diverticulitis, diverticulosis).
- Gallstones
- Elevated cholesterol levels from whatever reasons including genetic predisposition and a higher fat diet. Regulate results in decreases in total and LDL levels without lowering HDL levels.
- Cardiovascular disease including hypertension and coronary artery disease
- Insulin resistance and diabetes.

Antiox

An advanced antioxidant blend that spares no effort or expense to bring you the best antioxidant protection available today.

Antiox is by far the best antioxidant on the market today. With its synergistic blend of powerful antioxidants Antiox provides targeted antioxidant protection to all tissues in the body including the musculoskeletal system and the liver.

Antiox contains the usual antioxidants (including beta-carotene, vitamins E and C, zinc and selenium), and it also contains higher-level (and more expensive) antioxidants and immune enhancers including glutathione, the most important, all-purpose, endogenous antioxidant in our bodies. Our brand of glutathione, unlike most, is absorbed from the GI tract and used both systemically in all tissues in the body but especially by the liver in its role as the primary detoxifying organ in the body.

As well, Antiox contains other potent antioxidants including lipoic acid, lycopene, resveratrol (from red wine) and grape seed extract.

MVM

MD+ MVM is a comprehensive, specially balanced, multiple vitamin and mineral formula, with added ingredients, designed to provide full spectrum nutrition to anyone who diets or exercises.

MVM is the most complete foundational nutritional supplement available for the special needs that the athlete has for body maintenance, recuperation and repair. MVM supplies all the basic nutrients that may be depleted in those who exercise and is formulated to complement all our other products.

Even with the best of diets, it's still possible to have some marginal deficiencies due to depleted soils, the overuse of chemical fertilizers and poor farming, processing, storage and transportation practices. Add that to the fact that most of us do not even eat a well-balanced diet every day, and you can see how important it is for everyone, and especially athletes, to use a high quality multiple vitamin/mineral supplement.

MVM contains a complete mix of all of the important, and more expensive, vitamins and minerals. You will not see a bloated ingredients list in MVM's nutrition panel. When you put out a high quality, high dosage, complete vitamin and mineral formula there is no need to use miniscule sprinklings of bran, kelp, wheat germ, bee pollen, rose hips, and various fruit and vegetable powders, just to give the consumer the impression that they are getting good value for their dollar.

JointSupport

A comprehensive formula for joint and muscle pain and inflammation, arthritis and sports injuries.

JointSupport is the premier muscle and joint formula in the World. JointSupport has marked anti-inflammatory and healing effects and is useful for treating muscle soreness, acute and chronic injuries and for injury prevention.

With its many ingredients, Joint Support decreases inflammation and maximizes muscle, connective tissue and cartilage repair and maintenance. Joint Support, with its 36 synergistic ingredients, offers much more than any other product on the market today.

JointSupport:

- Protects joints and other tissues from the effects of excessive exercise and oxidant damage.
- Provides the ingredients the body needs for the maintenance and repair of joints, ligaments, tendons and muscle.
- Decreases inflammation, muscle irritability and spasm, swelling and pain, and helps heal sore and injured muscle, tendons, ligaments and joints.
- Supports the anabolic and anticatabolic hormones and processes that increase recovery and healing.
- Decreases natural wear and tear on the body, musculoskeletal system and skin.
- Bolsters the immune system

Besides all the ingredients targeted for the relief of inflammation, muscle and joint pain, and maintenance and repair of musculoskeletal tissues, JointSupport also contains the cutting edge, exclusive, patented, and highly bioavailable, **Biocell Collagen II** (BC-II). BC-II is the most comprehensive and advanced ingredient for joint support. But that is not all. BC-II has also been shown to relieve musculoskeletal pain in various conditions including arthritis and fibromyalgia, and to enhance skin health and elasticity resulting in younger, healthier looking skin.

BOTTOM LINE

JointSupport is the perfect solution for maintaining a healthy, pain free body and dealing with the aftermath of strenuous physical exercise.

Power Drink

Advanced Anabolic, AntiCatabolic, Fat Burning Training Drink

Power Drink fills a gap that is been overlooked by all the other supplement companies. While they are absorbed in what to use before and after training,

and rightly so, they are missing one of the most important opportunities for maximizing the results you get from training.

We all know that during training muscle is broken down. Most people believe that this breakdown is a necessary part of training. After all you have to break muscle tissue down before you can build it up. Do not you? Unfortunately that is one of the most stubborn training myths. Muscle breakdown isn't what provides the adaptation stimulus for increasing muscle size. It's the damage done to the muscle cell structure and the subsequent adaptation to that damage that determines the muscle building response. You do not have to break down the muscle at all to get this response in full force. In fact doing so is counter productive. The more muscle you keep from breaking down, and the more you increase protein synthesis, the better the results from your training. Taking Power Drink while you are training will put you miles ahead of everyone else who just uses water or at best a carbohydrate, low protein drink.

Power Drink, because of its effects on increasing protein synthesis and decreasing protein breakdown, is a powerful anabolic and anticatabolic product. As well, Power Drink increases cellular hydration and the utilization of amino acids and creatine by working muscle. As if that wasn't enough, Power Drink, because of its positive effects on the fat burning hormones and mechanisms actually allows you to burn more bodyfat while you are training. And with the other ingredients included in Power Drink you can train harder and longer and know that you have a powerful ally that will help you make good use of all that hard work.

Bottom line is that Power Drink is a revolutionary new concept in training drinks. This drink provides the nutrients necessary to increase muscle size and decrease bodyfat. By providing all the necessary ingredients to feed working muscles and shift the use of bodyfat as the energy source for training, Power Drink dramatically increases the positive effects of training, allows you train longer and harder, and increases recovery.
Power Drink is ideal for both those who want to increase muscle size and lose bodyfat and those who simply want to lose weight and bodyfat but maintain the muscle they now have.

Besides the hefty dose (44 grams) of the best quality proteins available anywhere, Power Drink also contains amino acids, electrolytes and other ingredients that will replace and replenish nutrients and fluid lost through exercise, prevent muscle cramps, and increase training time and efficiency.

There is no other product on the market anywhere in the world like Power Drink.

Metabolic

Advanced Anabolic and Fat Loss Primer

Metabolic normalizes and optimizes metabolism and macronutrient utilization (the use of fats, carbs and protein). It also has significant effects on the body's hormonal balance. It increases levels of growth hormone and testosterone (in both men and women), decreases cortisol levels, increases insulin sensitivity, and optimizes thyroid hormone levels and function. These effects increase weight and fat loss while maintaining or even increasing muscle mass. As well, the hormonal environment created by Metabolic will allow cellulite, that stubborn dimpled fat, to be oxidized along with the rest of the bodyfat.

The ingredients in Metabolic function synergistically to increase the anabolic and fat burning effects of exercise, and to combat fatigue, wear and tear on the body, stress and hormonal dysfunction.

Creatine Advantage

The Ultimate Creatine Product, With Several Synergistic Ingredients Meant to Maximize the Body's Energy Systems.

So advanced that it's being copied, but never duplicated, by the major supplement companies.

Creatine Advantage maximizes and enhances the anabolic and energy enhancing effects of creatine. It's the most advanced, and copied, creatine formula on the market today.

While creatine monohydrate has been shown to enhance athletic performance, and to increase strength and muscle mass, these effects are enhanced in Creatine Advantage by stacking creatine with other ingredients. Our formula not only contains the highest quality, pure crystalline creatine monohydrate so that it mixes instantly and leave's no chalky taste, but we have also added a host of other natural ingredients to give our formula an advantage over all other creatine products on the market.

Added amino acids and dipeptides and other essential boosters allow an increase in the absorption and utilization of creatine and increase the volumizing, anticatabolic and anabolic effect of the formula. The added energy ingredients and precursors make Creatine Advantage the ultimate creatine and energy mix, one that will maximize muscle mass and performance.

Unlike many other "advanced" creatine products, Creatine Advantage is based on real science and my expertise instead of hype and false promises.

It has a low carbohydrate based insulin boosting system (glutamine in the form of glutamine peptides – more stable in liquid form and more effective than free glutamine) and compounds to increase insulin sensitivity (chromium, taurine – which also has significant antioxidant and protective effects, stimulates growth hormone secretion and increases cell volume, and alpha lipoic acid – which is also an excellent antioxidant) and thus make the insulin more effective.

It also contains all the necessary products for the synthesis of both high energy phosphate compounds creatine phosphate and ATP, and for the efficient salvage of ATP after it's been metabolically degraded, including:

- The inorganic phosphorus and phosphates – also important for normalizing and regulating thyroid hormone;
- Creatine;
- Inosine;
- Ribose.

On top of that Creatine Advantage contains:

1. **Glutamine peptides**, which have anabolic (increases protein synthesis and muscle mass) and anticatabolic (decrease muscle breakdown) effects, above those normally associated with glutamine, as the peptides themselves have some physiological effects. Also the peptide form is better absorbed than free glutamine that is not peptide bonded.

   As well, the glutamine in the glutamine peptides:

   - Regulates protein synthesis;
   - Increases both aerobic and anaerobic energy systems;
   - Has beneficial effects on the immune system;
   - Aids in the prevention and treatment of the overtraining syndrome.

2. **Nutrients to facilitate the glycolytic and TCA cycle energy processes**:

   - **Biotin** – a cofactor in many energy reactions involving glycolytic, TCA and anapleurotic enzymes.
   - **Magnesium** – which has also been shown to increase energy systems, insulin sensitivity, protein synthesis and serum testosterone, GH and IGF-I levels.

- **Calcium** – which has been shown to facilitate muscle contraction and decreasing fatigue).
- **Potassium** – the transport of which is linked to aerobic glycolysis.

3. **An advanced cell volumizing (resulting in increases in protein synthesis and an anabolic effect) formula containing**

- Glutamine;
- Taurine;
- Potassium;
- Sodium;
- Creatine (which has significant volumizing effects).

References

1. Westman EC, Yancy WS, Edman JS, Tomlin KF, Perkins CE. Effect of 6-month adherence to a very low carbohydrate diet program. Am J Med 2002 Jul;113(1):30-6.

2. Judd JT, Baer DJ, Clevidence BA, Kris-Etherton P, Muesing RA, Iwane M. Dietary cis and trans monounsaturated and saturated FA and plasma lipids and lipoproteins in men. Lipids 2002; 37(2):123-31.

3. Smith DR, Wood R, Tseng S, Smith SB. Increased beef consumption increases apolipoprotein A-I but not serum cholesterol of mildly hypercholesterolemic men with different levels of habitual beef intake. Exp Biol Med (Maywood) 2002; 227(4):266-75.

4. Parks EJ, Krauss RM, Hellerstein MK, et al. Effects of a low-fat, high-carbohydrate diet on VLDL-triglyceride assembly, production, and clearance. J Clin Invest 1999;104:1087–95.

5. Volek JS, Sharman MJ, Love DM, Avery NG, Gomez AL, Scheett TP, Kraemer WJ. Body composition and hormonal responses to a carbohydrate-restricted diet. Metabolism 2002 Jul;51(7):864-70.

6. Young CM, Scanlan SS, Im HS, Lutwak L. Effect on body composition and other parameters in obese young men of carbohydrate level of reduction diet. Am J Clin Nutr 1971; 24:290-296.

7. Willi SM, Oexmann MJ, Wright NM, Collop NA, Key LL Jr. The effects of a high-protein, low-fat, ketogenic diet on adolescents with morbid obesity: body composition, blood chemistries, and sleep abnormalities. Pediatrics 1998; 101:61-67.

8. Nemeth PM, Rosser BW, Choksi RM, Norris BJ, Baker KM. Metabolic response to a high-fat diet in neonatal and adult rat muscle. American Journal of Physiology 1992; 262(2 Pt 1):C282-6.

9. Reynolds AJ, Fuhrer L, Dunlap HL, Finke M, Kallfelz FA. Effect of diet and training on muscle glycogen storage and utilization in sled dogs. J Appl Physiol 1995 Nov;79(5):1601-7.

10. Boyadjiev N. Increase of aerobic capacity by submaximal training and high-fat diets. Folia Med (Plovdiv) 1996;38(1):49-59.

11. Conlee RK, Hammer RL, Winder WW, et al. Glycogen depletion and exercise in rats adapted to a high fat diet. Metabolism 1990: 39(3):289-94.

[12] Nakamura M, Brown J, Miller WC. Glycogen depletion patterns in trained rats adapted to a high-fat or high-carbohydrate diet. Int J Sports Med 1998 Aug;19(6):419-24.

[13] Lambert EV, Speechly DP, Dennis SC, and Noakes TD. Enhanced endurance in trained cyclists during moderate intensity exercise following 2 weeks adaptation to a high fat diet. Eur J Appl Physiol 69: 287-293, 1994.

[14] Rowlands DS, Hopkins WG. Effects of high-fat and high-carbohydrate diets on metabolism and performance in cycling. Metabolism 2002 Jun;51(6):678-90.

[15] Helge JW, Ayre K, Chaunchaiyakul S, Hulbert AJ, Kiens B, Storlien LH. Endurance in high-fat-fed rats: effects of carbohydrate content and fatty acid profile. J Appl Physiol 1998 Oct;85(4):1342-8.

[16] Pogliaghi S, Veicsteinas A. Influence of low and high dietary fat on physical performance in untrained males. Med Sci Sports Exerc 1999 Jan;31(1):149-55.

[17] Helge JW. Adaptation to a fat-rich diet: effects on endurance performance in humans. Sports Med 2000 Nov;30(5):347-57.

[18] Lapachet RA, Miller WC, Arnall DA. Bodyfat and exercise endurance in trained rats adapted to a high-fat and/or high-carbohydrate diet. J Appl Physiol 1996 Apr;80(4):1173-9.

[19] Carey AL, Staudacher HM, Cummings NK, Stepto NK, Nikolopoulos V, Burke LM, Hawley JA. Effects of fat adaptation and carbohydrate restoration on prolonged endurance exercise. J Appl Physiol 2001 Jul;91(1):115-22.

[20] Lambert EV, Hawley JA, Goedecke J, Noakes TD, Dennis SC. Nutritional strategies for promoting fat utilization and delaying the onset of fatigue during prolonged exercise. J Sports Sci 1997 Jun;15(3):315-24.

[21] Pitsiladis YP, Smith I, Maughan RJ. Increased fat availability enhances the capacity of trained individuals to perform prolonged exercise. Med Sci Sports Exerc 1999 Nov;31(11):1570-9.

[22] Goldin BR, Woods MN, Spiegelman DL, et al. The effect of dietary fat and fiber on serum estrogen concentrations in premenopausal women under controlled dietary conditions. Cancer 1994; 74(3 Suppl):1125-31.

[23] Lavoie JM, Helie R, Peronnet F, Cousineau D, Provencher PJ. Effects of muscle CHO-loading manipulations on hormonal responses during prolonged exercise. International Journal of Sports Medicine 1985; 6(2):95-9.

[24] Schurch PM, Hillen M, Hock A, Feinendegen LE, Hollmann W. Possibilities of calculating the fat-free body mass and its reaction to a carbohydrate-poor, fat-rich diet. Infusionstherapie und Klinische Ernahrung 1979; 6(5):311-4.

[25] Kather H, Wieland E, Scheurer A, et al. Influences of variation in total energy intake and dietary composition on regulation of fat cell lipolysis in ideal weight subjects. J Clin Invest 1987; 80(2):566-72.

[26] Rabast U, Kasper H, Schonborn J. Comparative studies in obese subjects fed carbohydrate-restricted and high carbohydrate 1,000-calorie formula diets. Nutr Metab 1978; 22(5):269-77.

[27] Flatt JP. Use and storage of carbohydrate and fat. [Review] American Journal of Clinical Nutrition 1995; 61(4 Suppl):952S-959S.

[28] Sandretto AM, Tsai AC. Effects of fat intake on body composition and hepatic lipogenic enzyme activities of hamsters shortly after exercise cessation. Amer J Clin Nutr 1988; 47(2): 175-9.

[29] Tsai AC, Gong TW. Modulation of the exercise and retirement effects by dietary fat intake in hamsters. J Nutr 1987; 117(6):1149-53.

[30] Thompson JR, Wu G. The effect of ketone bodies on nitrogen metabolism in skeletal muscle. Comp Biochem Physiol 1991; 100(2):209-16.

[31] Ohtsuka A, Hayashi K, Noda T, Tomita Y. Reduction of corticosterone-induced muscle proteolysis and growth retardation by a combined treatment with insulin, testosterone and high protein-high-fat diet in rats. J Nutr Sci Vitaminol 1992; 38(1):83-92.

[32] McCarger LJ, Baracos VE and Clandinin MT. Influence of dietary carbohydrate-to-fat ratio on whole body nitrogen retention and body composition in adult rats. J Nutr 1989; 119(9):1240-5.

[33] Magistretti PJ, Pellerin L. [Functional brain imaging: role metabolic coupling between astrocytes and neurons]. Rev Med Suisse Romande 2000 Sep;120(9):739-42.

[34] Deitmer JW. Strategies for metabolic exchange between glial cells and neurons. Respir Physiol 2001 Dec;129(1-2):71-81.

[35] Ingram DM, Bennett FC, Willcox D, de Klerk N. Effect of low-fat diet on female sex hormone levels. J Nat Cancer Inst 1987; 79(6):1225-9.

[36] Sebokova E, Garg ML, Wierzbicki A, et al. Alteration of the lipid composition of rat testicular plasma membranes by dietary (n-3) fatty acids changes the responsiveness of Leydig cells and testosterone synthesis. J Nutr 1990; 120(6):610-18.

[37] Campbell WW, Barton ML Jr, Cyr-Campbell D, Davey SL, Beard JL, Parise G, Evans WJ. Effects of an omnivorous diet compared with a lacto-ovo vegetarian diet on resistance-training-induced changes in body composition and skeletal muscle in older men. Am J Clin Nutr 1999 Dec;70(6):1032-9.

[38] Fossati P. Fontaine P. Endocrine and metabolic consequences of massive obesity. Revue du Praticien 1993; 43(15):1935-9.

[39] Schurch PM, Reinke A, Hollmann W. Carbohydrate-reduced diet and metabolism: about the influence of a 4-week isocaloric fat-rich, carbohydrate-reduced diet on body weight and metabolism. Medizinische Klinik-Munich 1979; 74(36):1279-85.

[40] Westman EC, Yancy WS, Edman JS, Tomlin KF, Perkins CE. Effect of 6-month adherence to a very low carbohydrate diet program. Am J Med 2002 Jul;113(1):30-6.

[41] Sidery MB, Gallen IW, Macdonald IA. The initial physiological responses to glucose ingestion in normal subjects are modified by a 3 day high-fat diet. Br J Nutr 1990; 64(3):705-13.

[42] Bhathena SJ, Berlin E, Judd JT, et al. Dietary fat and menstrual-cycle effects on the erythrocyte ghost insulin receptor in premenopausal women. Am J Clin Nutr 1989; 50(3):460-4.

[43] Burke LM, Angus DJ, Cox GR, Cummings NK, Febbraio MA, Gawthorn K, Hawley JA, Minehan M, Martin DT, Hargreaves M. Effect of fat adaptation and carbohydrate restoration on metabolism and performance during prolonged cycling. J Appl Physiol 2000 Dec;89(6):2413-

[44] Carey AL, Staudacher HM, Cummings NK, Stepto NK, Nikolopoulos V, Burke LM, Hawley JA. Effects of fat adaptation and carbohydrate restoration on prolonged endurance exercise. J Appl Physiol 2001 Jul;91(1):115-22.

[45] Kather H, Wieland E, Scheurer A, et al. Influences of variation in total energy intake and dietary composition on regulation of fat cell lipolysis in ideal-weight subjects. J Clin Inv 1987; 80(2):566-72.

[46] Goodman MN, Lowell B, Belur E, Ruderman NB. Sites of protein conservation and loss during starvation: influence of adiposity. American Journal of Physiology 1984; 246(5 Pt 1):E383-90.

[47] Liu S, Baracos VE, Quinney HA, Clandinin MT. Dietary omega-3 and polyunsaturated fatty acids modify fatty acyl composition and insulin binding in skeletal-muscle sarcolemma. Biochemical Journal 1994; 299(Pt 3):831-837.

[48] Kruger MC. Eicosapentaenoic acid and docosahexaenoic acid supplementation increases calcium balance. Nutrition Research 1995;15;211-219.

[49] Ip C, Singh M, Thompson HJ, Scimeca JA. Conjugated linoleic acid suppresses mammary carcinogenesis and proliferative activity of the mammary gland in the rat. Cancer Research 1994; 54(5):1212-5.

[50] Ip C, Scimeca JA, Thompson HJ. Conjugated linoleic acid. A powerful anticarcinogen from animal fat sources. [Review] Cancer 1994; 74(3 Suppl):1050-4.

[51] Pariza MW. Ha YL. Benjamin H. Sword JT. Gruter A. Chin SF. Storkson J. Faith N. Albright K. Formation and action of anticarcinogenic fatty acids. [Review] Advances in Experimental Medicine & Biology. 289:269-72, 1991.

[52] Shultz TD, Chew BP, Seaman WR, Luedecke LO. Inhibitory effect of conjugated dienoic derivatives of linoleic acid and beta-carotene on the in vitro growth of human cancer cells. Cancer Letters 1992; 63(2):125-33.

[53] Hodgson JM, Wahlqvist ML, Boxall JA, Lalazs ND. Can linoleic acid contribute to coronary artery disease? Am J Clin Nutr 1993; 58(2):228-34.

[54] Davidson MH. Implications for the present and direction for the future. Am J Card 1993; 71(6):32B-36B.

[55] Ni JS, Wu JX, Xiao RQ. [The preventive and curative action of fish oil compound on early atherosclerotic lesions in the aortic of diabetic rats]. Chung-Hua Ping Li Hsueh Tsa Chih – Chinese Journal of Pathology 1994; 23(1):31-3.

[56] Henzen C. Fish oil-healing principle in the Eskimo Diet? Schweizerische Rundschau fur Medizin Praxis 1995; 84(1):11-15.

[57] Artemis P Simopoulos. Essential fatty acids in health and chronic disease. American Journal of Clinical Nutrition, Vol. 70, No. 3, 560S-569S, September 1999.

[58] Garg ML, Wierzbicki A, Keelan M, Thomson AB, Clandinin MT. Fish oil prevents change in arachidonic acid and cholesterol content in rat caused by dietary cholesterol. Lipids 1989; 24(4):266-70.

[59] Schurch PM, Reinke A, Hollmann W. Carbohydrate-reduced diet and metabolism: about the influence of a 4-week isocaloric, fat-rich, carbohydrate-reduced diet on body weight and metabolism [Review]. Medizinische Klinik-Muich 1979; 74(36):1279-85.

[60] Awad AB, Zepp EA. Alteration of rat adipose tissue lipolytic response to norepinephrine by dietary fatty acid manipulation. Biochem Biophys Res Comm 1979; 86:138-144.

[61] Parrish CC, Pathy DA, Parkes JG, Angel A. Dietary fish oils modify adipocyte structure and function. J Cell Phys 1991; 148(3):493-502.

[62] Belzung F, Raclot T, Groscolas R. Fish oil n-3 fatty acids selectively limit the hypertrophy of abdominal fat depots in growing fats fed high-fat diets. Am J Physiol 1993; 264(6 Pt 2): R1111-R1118.

[63] Parrish CC, Pathy DA, Angel A. Dietary fish oils limit adipose tissue hypertrophy in rats. Metabolism: Clin Exp 1990; 39(3):217-19.

[64] Barham JB, Edens MB, Fonteh AN, Johnson MM, Easter L, Chilton FH. Addition of eicosapentaenoic acid to gamma-linolenic acid-supplemented diets prevents serum arachidonic acid accumulation in humans. J Nutr 2000 Aug;130(8):1925-31.

[65] Vasil'ev AV, Samsonov MA, Pokrovskii VB, Pokrovskaia GR, Levachev MM. [Characteristics of the humoral immune system and lipid peroxidation processes in people living in territories contaminated with radionuclides]. Voprosy Meditsinskoi Khimii 1994; 40(2):21-4.

[66] Volgarev MN, Levachev MM, Trushchina EN, et al. [The modulation of the function of the immunocompetent system and of nonspecific body resistance in rats with different ratios of essential fatty acids in the diet]. Byulleten Eksperimentalnoi Biologii i Meditsiny 1993; 116(12):607-9

[67] Razzini E, Baronzio GF. Omega-3 fatty acids as coadjuvant treatment in AIDS. [Review] Medical Hypotheses 1993; 41(4):300-5.

[68] Philip W, James T, Ralph A. Dietary fats and cancer. Nutr Res 1992; 12(SUPPL):S147-S158.

[69] Lichtenstein AH, Ausman LM, Carrasco W, et al. Effects of canola, corn, and olive oils on fasting and postprandial plasma lipoproteins in humans as part of a National Cholesterol Education Program Step 2 diet. Arteriosclerosis & Thrombosis 1993; 13(10):1533-42.

[70] Willett WC, Stampfer MJ, Manson JE, et. al. Intake of trans fatty acids and risk of coronary heart disease among women. Lancet 1993; 341(8845):581-5.

[71] Mensink RP, Zock PL, Katan MB, Hornstra G. Effect of dietary cis and trans fatty acids on serum lipoprotein[a] levels in humans. Journal of Lipid Research 1992; 33(10):1493-501.

[72] Booyens J, Louwrens CC, Katzeff IE. The Eskimo diet. Prophylactic effects ascribed to the balanced presence of natural cis unsaturated fatty acids and to the absence of unnatural trans and cis isomers of unsaturated fatty acids. Medical Hypotheses 1986; 21(4):387-408.

[73] Mantzioris E, James MJ, Gibson RA, Cleland LG. Differences exist in the relationships between dietary linoleic and alpha-linolenic acids and their respective long-chain metabolites. American Journal of Clinical Nutrition 1995; 61(2):320-4.

[74] Kobayashi J, Yokoyama S, Kitamura S. Eicosapentaenoic acid modulates arachidonic acid metabolism in rat alveolar macrophages. Prostaglandins Leukot Essent Fatty Acids 1995; 52(4):259-62.

[75] Taouis M, Dagou C, Ster C, Durand G, Pinault M, Delarue J. N-3 polyunsaturated fatty acids prevent the defect of insulin receptor signaling in muscle. Am J Physiol Endocrinol Metab 2002 Mar;282(3):E664-71.

[76] Bartram HP, Gostner A, Scheppach W, et al. Effects of fish oil on rectal cell proliferation, mucosal fatty acids, and prostaglandin E2 release in healthy subjects. Gastroenterology 1993; 105(5):1317-22.

[77] Rose DP, Connolly JM, Rayburn J, Coleman M. Influence of diets containing eicosapentaenoic or docosahexaenoic acid on growth and metastasis of breast cancer cells in nude mice. J Natl Cancer Inst 1995; 87(8):587-92.

[78] Curtis CL, Hughes CE, Flannery CR, Little CB, Harwood JL, Caterson B. n-3 fatty acids specifically modulate catabolic factors involved in articular cartilage degradation. *J Biol Chem* 2000 Jan 14;275(2):721-4.

[79] Tomobe YI, Morizawa K, Tsuchida M, Hibino H, Nakano Y, Tanaka Y. Dietary docosahexaenoic acid suppresses inflammation and immunoresponses in contact hypersensitivity reaction in mice. *Lipids* 2000 Jan;35(1):61-9.

[80] Ascherio A, Rimm EB, Stampfer MJ, Giovannucci EL, Willett WC. Dietary intake of marine n-3 fatty acids, fish intake, and the risk of coronary disease among men. N Engl J Med 1995; 332(15):977-82.

[81] von Schacky C. n-3 fatty acids and the prevention of coronary atherosclerosis. *Am J Clin Nutr* 2000 Jan;71(1 Suppl):224S-7S.

[82] Eritsland J, Arnesen H, Seljeflot I, Hostmark AT. Long-term metabolic effects of n-3 polyunsaturated fatty acids in patients with coronary artery disease. Am J Clin Nutr 1995; 61(4):831-6.

[83] Wahrburg U, Martin H, Sandkamp M, Schulte H, Assmann G. Comparative effects of a recommended lipid-lowering diet vs a diet rich in monounsaturated fatty acids on serum lipid profiles in healthy young adults. Am J Clin Nutr 1992; 56(4):678-83.

[84] Lichtenstein AH, Ausman LM, Carrasco W, et al. Rice bran oil consumption and plasma lipid levels in moderately hypercholesterolemic humans. Arteriosclerosis & Thrombosis 1994; 14(4):549-56.

[85] Keys A, Menotti A, Karvonen MJ, et al. The diet and 15-year death rate in the seven countries study. Am J Epidemiol 1986; 124(6):903-15.

[86] Katsouyanni K, Skalkidis Y, Petridou E, et al. Diet and peripheral arterial occlusive disease: the role of poly-, mono-, and saturated fatty acids. Am J Epidemiol 1991; 133(1):24-31.

[87] Aviram M, Eias K. Dietary olive oil reduces low-density lipoprotein uptake by macrophages and decreases the susceptibility of the lipoprotein to undergo lipid peroxidation. Annals of Nutrition & Metabolism 1993; 37(2):75-84.

[88] Massaro M, Carluccio MA, De Caterina R. Direct vascular antiatherogenic effects of oleic acid: a clue to the cardioprotective effects of the Mediterranean diet. Cardiologia 1999 Jun;44(6):507-13.

[89] Vissers MN, Zock PL, Roodenburg AJ, Leenen R, Katan MB. Olive oil phenols are absorbed in humans. J Nutr 2002 Mar;132(3):409-17.

[90] Leenen R, Roodenburg AJ, Vissers MN, Schuurbiers JA, van Putte KP, Wiseman SA, van de Put FH. Supplementation of plasma with olive oil phenols and extracts: influence on LDL oxidation. J Agric Food Chem 2002 Feb 27;50(5):1290-7.

[91] McNamara DJ. Dietary fatty acids, lipoproteins, and cardiovascular disease. [Review] Adv Food Nutr Res 1992; 36:253-351.

[92] Denke MA. Grundy SM. Effects of fats high in stearic acid on lipid and lipoprotein concentrations in men [see comments]. Am J Clin Nutr 1991; 54(6):1036-40.

[93] Katan MB. Zock PL. Mensink RP. Effects of fats and fatty acids on blood lipids in humans: an overview. [Review] Am J Clin Nutr 1994; 60(6 Suppl):1017S-1022S.

[94] Hansen JC, Pedersen HS, Mulvad G. Fatty acids and antioxidants in the Inuit diet. Their role in ischemic heart disease (IHD) and possible interactions with other dietary factors. A review. Arctic Medical Research 1994; 53(1):4-17.

[95] A Chesley, JD MacDougall, MA Tarnopolsky et al., "Changes in muscle protein synthesis after resistance exercise," J Appl Physiol 73 (1992): 1383-1388.

[96] Gardi J, Obal F Jr, Fang J, Zhang J, Krueger JM. Diurnal variations and sleep deprivation-induced changes in rat hypothalamic GHRH and somatostatin contents. Am J Physiol 1999 Nov;277(5 Pt 2):R1339-R1344.

[97] Van Cauter E, Copinschi G. Interrelationships between growth hormone and sleep. Growth Horm IGF Res 2000 Apr;10 Suppl B:S57-62.

[98] Youngstedt SD, O'Connor PJ, Dishman RK. The effects of acute exercise on sleep: a quantitative synthesis. Sleep 1997 Mar;20(3):203-14.

99 Gambelunghe C, Rossi R, Mariucci G, Tantucci M, Ambrosini MV. Effects of light physical exercise on sleep regulation in rats. Med Sci Sports Exerc 2001 Jan;33(1):57-60.

100 Kubitz KA, Landers DM, Petruzzello SJ, Han M. The effects of acute and chronic exercise on sleep. A meta-analytic review. Sports Med 1996 Apr;21(4):277-91.

101 Driver S, Taylor SR. Sleep disturbances and exercise. Sports Med 1996 Jan;21(1):1-6.

102 Van Cauter E. Slow wave sleep and release of growth hormone. JAMA 2000 Dec 6;284(21):2717-8.

103 Luboshitzky R, Herer P, Levi M, Shen-Orr Z, Lavie P. Relationship between rapid eye movement sleep and testosterone secretion in normal men. J Androl 1999 Nov-Dec;20(6):731-7.

104 Nindl BC, Hymer WC, Deaver DR, Kraemer WJ. Growth hormone pulsatility profile characteristics following acute heavy resistance exercise. J Appl Physiol 2001 Jul;91(1):163-172.

105 Kern W, Perras B, Wodick R, Fehm HL, Born J. Hormonal secretion during nighttime sleep indicating stress of daytime exercise. J Appl Physiol 1995 Nov;79(5):1461-8.

106 Dijk DJ, Duffy JF, Czeisler CA. Contribution of circadian physiology and sleep homeostasis to age-related changes in human sleep. Chronobiol Int 2000 May;17(3):285-311.

107 Van Cauter E, Leproult R, Plat L. Age-related changes in slow wave sleep and REM sleep and relationship with growth hormone and cortisol levels in healthy men. JAMA 2000 Aug 16;284(7):861-8. Comment in: JAMA. 2000 Aug 16;284(7):879-81

108 Haussinger D. Control of protein turnover by the cellular hydratation state. Ital J Gastroenterol 1993 Jan;25(1):42-8.

109 Waldegger S, Busch GL, Kaba NK, Zempel G, Ling H, Heidland A, Haussinger D, Lang F. Effect of cellular hydration on protein metabolism. Miner Electrolyte Metab 1997;23(3-6):201-5.

110 Uthgenannt D, Schoolmann D, Pietrowsky R, Fehm HL, Born J. Effects of sleep on the production of cytokines in humans. Psychosom Med 1995 Mar-Apr;57(2):97-104.

111 Piatti PM, Monti LD, Pacchioni M, Pontiroli AE, Pozza G. Forearm insulin- and non-insulin-mediated glucose uptake and muscle metabolism in man: role of free fatty acids and blood glucose levels. Metabolism: Clinical & Experimental 1991; 40(9):926-33.

112 Felig P, Wahren J, Sherwin R, Palaiologos G. Amino acid and protein metabolism in diabetes mellitus. Archives of Internal Medicine 1977; 137(4):507-13.

[113] Favier RJ, Koubi HE, Mayet MH, Sempore B, Simi B, Flandrois R. Effects of gluconeogenic precursor flux alterations on glycogen resynthesis. after prolonged exercise. J Appl Physiol 1987; 63(5)p1733-8.

[114] Azzout B, Bois-Joyeux B, Chanez M, Peret J. Development of gluconeogenesis from various precursors in isolated rat hepatocytes during starvation or after feeding a high protein, carbohydrate-free diet. Journal of Nutrition 1987; 117(1):164-9.

[115] Jahoor F, Peters EJ, Wolfe RR. The relationship between gluconeogenic substrate supply and glucose production in humans. American Journal of Physiology 1990; 258(2 Pt 1):E288-96.